Fast Facts

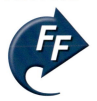

Fast Facts: Chronic and Cancer Pain

Fourth edition

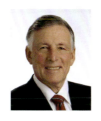

Michael J Cousins AO MD DSc FFPMANZCA FRCA
FANZCA FAChPM(RACP) FAICD FFPMCA(Hon)
DSc(Hon McMaster) FAHMS(Hon)
Emeritus Professor and Head
Pain Management Research Institute
Royal North Shore Hospital (Retired)
Kolling Institute, University of Sydney
New South Wales, Australia

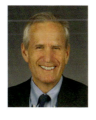

Rollin M Gallagher MD MPH DABPM FAAPM FAPA
Editor-in-Chief, *Pain Medicine*
Clinical Professor of Psychiatry and Anesthesiology
 Director for Health Policy Research and Primary Care
 Penn Pain Medicine, University of Pennsylvania
Consultant, Pain Management Work Group
 Health Executive Council,
 Departments of Defense and Veterans Affairs
Philadelphia, USA

Declaration of Independence
This book is as balanced and as practical as we ca
Ideas for improvement are always welcome: feedb

HEALTH PRESS

Fast Facts: Chronic and Cancer Pain
First published 2007; second edition 2011; third edition 2015
Fourth edition June 2017

Text © 2017 Michael J Cousins, Rollin M Gallagher
© 2017 in this edition Health Press Limited

Health Press Limited, Elizabeth House, Queen Street, Abingdon,
Oxford OX14 3LN, UK
Tel: +44 (0)1235 523233

Book orders can be placed by telephone or via the website.
To order via the website, please go to: fastfacts.com
For telephone orders, please call +44 (0)1752 202301.

Fast Facts is a trademark of Health Press Limited.

All rights reserved. No part of this publication may be reproduced, stored in a retrieval system, or transmitted in any form or by any means, electronic, mechanical, photocopying, recording or otherwise, without the express permission of the publisher.

The rights of Michael J Cousins and Rollin M Gallagher to be identified as the authors of this work have been asserted in accordance with the Copyright, Designs & Patents Act 1988 Sections 77 and 78.

The publisher and the authors have made every effort to ensure the accuracy of this book, but cannot accept responsibility for any errors or omissions.

For all drugs, please consult the product labeling approved in your country for prescribing information.

Registered names, trademarks, etc. used in this book, even when not marked as such, are not to be considered unprotected by law.

A CIP record for this title is available from the British Library.

ISBN 978-1-910797-35-8

Cousins MJ (Michael)
Fast Facts: Chronic and Cancer Pain/
Michael J Cousins, Rollin M Gallagher

Medical illustrations by Annamaria Dutto, Beverley, UK.
Printed in China with Xpedient Print.

List of abbreviations	4
Introduction	5
Definitions and mechanisms	7
Assessment of pain	30
Treatment options	47
Trigeminal neuralgia	73
Complex regional pain syndrome	79
Diabetic and postherpetic neuropathic pain	92
Central pain	106
Persistent postsurgical pain	117
Cancer pain	126
Musculoskeletal pain	137
Visceral pain	166
Headache	174
Acknowledgments and useful resources	185
Index	188

List of abbreviations

AMPA: alpha-amino-3-hydroxy-5-methyl-4-isoxazole propionic acid (receptor)

ASA: acetylsalicylic acid (aspirin)

ASIC: acid-sensing ion channel

BDNF: brain-derived neurotropic factor

BRM: biological response modifier

CBT: cognitive behavioral therapy

CNS: central nervous system

COX-2: cyclooxygenase-2 (inhibitor)

CPH: chronic paroxysmal hemicrania

CPSP: central post-stroke pain

CRPS: complex regional pain syndrome

CSF: cerebrospinal fluid

CT: computed tomography

DMARD: disease-modifying antirheumatic drug

DN: diabetic neuropathy

DNA: deoxyribonucleic acid

ECAP: evoked compound action potential

GABA: gamma-aminobutyric acid

HRQoL: health-related quality of life

IASP: International Association for the Study of Pain

IBS: irritable bowel syndrome

IL: interleukin

ISDA: intraspinal drug administration

MRI: magnetic resonance imaging

MS: multiple sclerosis

MVD: microvascular decompression

NK1: neurokinin-1 (receptor)

NMDA: N-methyl D-aspartate (receptor)

NNT: number needed to treat (for a positive outcome in one individual)

NO: nitric oxide

NRI: noradrenaline-reuptake inhibitor

NSAID: non-steroidal anti-inflammatory drug

PHN: postherpetic neuralgia

PKC: protein kinase C

PNS: peripheral nervous system/ peripheral nerve stimulation

PPSP: persistent postsurgical pain

RCT: randomized controlled trial

SAARD: slow-acting antirheumatic drug

SCI: spinal cord injury

SCS: spinal cord stimulation

SIP: sympathetically independent pain

SMP: sympathetically maintained pain

SNRI: serotonin–norepinephrine-reuptake inhibitor

SNS: sacral nerve stimulation

SSRI: selective serotonin-reuptake inhibitor

TCA: tricyclic antidepressant

TENS: transcutaneous electrical nerve stimulation

TNF: tumor necrosis factor

TRPV: transient receptor potential vanilloid (receptor)

VZV: varicella zoster virus

Introduction

On average, at least 1 in 5 people has chronic pain, with 30% being severely disabled by it. *All* clinicians, regardless of specialty, will see patients with pain that has persisted for more than 6 months, and this book is aimed at the wide range of busy health professionals who may be well aware they have received little education and training to help them manage such patients. The extraordinary situation where such a book is necessary has come about as a result of major ongoing deficiencies in pain education and training, the result of which is highlighted by the recent epidemic of overdoses amongst patients prescribed opioid analgesics.

There is growing awareness of the devastating effect that chronic pain has on individuals and their families, on society as a whole and on the economy in terms of lost output and productivity. The Global Burden of Disease Study 2013 revealed that low back pain was a leading cause of 'years lived with disability' in both 1990 and 2013. It is no wonder that many national governments now recognize chronic pain as a chronic 'condition', or more appropriately as a chronic disease. In fact, governments around the world are accepting the importance of developing specialized strategies for the prevention, treatment and management of chronic pain as a fundamental human right, and passing laws and regulations that encourage, and even mandate, improved systems of care for pain (see Key references, page 6).

Medical science has progressed from marginalizing chronic pain as merely a symptom of disease to developing a better understanding of its causes, effects and pathophysiological mechanisms, leading to new treatments aimed at a wide range of novel targets. New and old treatments are being integrated into comprehensive multimodal management plans focused on the control of pain, with the ultimate aim of improving function and quality of life.

This book describes a variety of chronic pain syndromes, and sets out the principles of assessment and treatment for each, with an eye toward successful early interventions that prevent pain chronification. It does not aim to be comprehensive. Rather, it seeks to distill a great deal of pain-related evidence and, because every individual's experience of pain is unique, we have adopted the current practice in clinical decision-making of 'evidence-guided' rather than 'evidence-based' medicine.

Assessment and treatment of chronic pain is most effectively carried out in a biopsychosocial framework, drawing on the knowledge and skills of a wide range of health professionals who need to work in an interdisciplinary manner. With health services around the world responding to calls to improve the management of painful long-term conditions, develop preventive and cost-effective solutions, respond to patient choice and voice, and create healthier workplaces, this is a timely resource that provides a concise introduction to the complex and extensive field of chronic pain for all health professionals wanting – and needing – to know more.

Key references

Global Burden of Disease Study 2013 Collaborators. Global, regional, and national incidence, prevalence, and years lived with disability for 301 acute and chronic diseases and injuries in 188 countries, 1990–2013: a systematic analysis for the Global Burden of Disease Study 2013. *Lancet* 2015;386:743–800.

Institute of Medicine (US) Committee on Advancing Pain Research, Care, and Education. *Relieving pain in America: a blueprint for transforming prevention, care, education, and research*. Washington (DC): National Academies Press, 2011. www.ncbi.nlm.nih.gov/books/NBK91497, last accessed 22 March 2017.

The Interagency Pain Research Coordinating Committee, Department of Health and Human Services. *National Pain Strategy: A Comprehensive Population Health-Level Strategy for Pain*, 18 March 2016. https://iprcc.nih.gov/docs/HHSNational_Pain_Strategy.pdf, last accessed 22 March 2017.

International Association for the Study of Pain. *Declaration of Montreal. Declaration that access to pain management is a fundamental human right*. www.iasp-pain.org/DeclarationofMontreal?navItemNumber=582 *Pain* 2011;152:2673-4, last accessed 22 March 2017.

Painaustralia. *National pain strategy: pain management for all Australians*. www.painaustralia.org.au/images/pain_australia/National%20Pain%20Strategy%202011%20Exec%20Summary.pdf, last accessed 22 March 2017.

1 Definitions and mechanisms

Defining pain

There are many ways to classify pain; for example, by duration, etiology or intensity (Table 1.1). As understanding of the cellular mechanisms of pain has increased, proposals have been advanced to classify pain according to the predominant pathophysiological mechanism thought to be involved.

Present-day pain research was heralded by the publication of Melzack and Wall's 'gate control theory' in 1965, which provided a model for the modulation of incoming nociceptive information by the central nervous

TABLE 1.1
Possible ways of classifying pain

By temporal pattern and duration
- Acute
- Subacute
- Chronic
- Episodic

By etiology
- Cancerous
- Ischemic
- Postoperative
- Injury

By intensity
- Mild
- Moderate
- Severe

By probable mechanism
- Tissue damage
- Inflammation
- Central sensitization of nociceptors
- Nerve-damage-triggered neuroplasticity changes
- Glia-derived neural sensitization
- Loss of inhibition
- Brain neuroplasticity changes
- 'Cross-talk' between sympathetic and sensory neurons

By type of injured tissue
- Nociceptive
- Neuropathic
- Visceral
- Somatic

system (CNS). After publication of that model, researchers never again viewed the peripheral nervous system (PNS) or CNS as collections of cables passively transmitting nociceptive information.

The nervous system is dynamic; it is plastic, in that its structure and function are shaped and reshaped by activity within it, and at each level it continually amplifies or inhibits the signals that the brain ultimately interprets as pain. This plasticity is fundamental to the understanding of both the perpetuation of pain in some pain syndromes and the mechanisms of action of pain treatment modalities. There is large variability in the neuroplasticity response among individuals, and this accounts for the large variability in pain response. For example, after surgery or trauma some patients suffer much higher than average acute pain levels. Importantly, these are the people who are at high risk of progression to persistent (chronic) pain.

Global health burden. Chronic pain is not tabulated as a separate diagnosis in the World Health Organization's comprehensive estimates of global health burdens associated with highly prevalent conditions. Yet it is through chronic pain that many of the greatest global health burdens – cancer, HIV/AIDS, diabetes, arthritis, alcoholism, drug abuse and trauma (including war) – exact their long-term human, social and economic toll. Mental health problems such as anxiety and depression also place sufferers at increased risk of developing chronic pain, while those with chronic pain are prone to develop new anxiety or depression.

Mechanisms of pain

It is universally recognized that factors in three domains contribute to the human experience of chronic pain: biological (nociceptive and neuropathic); psychological; and social (environmental). In fact, all three domains almost certainly exert their influence at various levels of the nervous system, with much overlap.

Biological. A stimulus of intensity sufficient to threaten tissue damage activates nociceptors, which are specialized nerve endings. A major advance has been the discovery of the process whereby noxious temperature (heat and cold) and chemical stimuli are detected and transduced into electrical energy and conducted along the axon to the spinal cord. The transduction process for the remaining category of noxious stimuli associated with pressure will likely soon be elucidated. Existing knowledge of temperature and chemical mechanisms includes the key role of transient receptor potential vanilloid (TRPV), acid-sensing ion channel (ASIC) and P_2X receptor sites, which have all become exciting new targets to block nociception at a peripheral level (Figure 1.1).

The cell bodies of these nociceptors (first-order neurons) are located outside the spinal cord in the dorsal root ganglia and extend their dendritic processes to the periphery. Activation of nociceptors triggers a volley of incoming impulses that travel to the spinal cord along both myelinated (Aδ) and unmyelinated (C) nerve fibers. These fibers enter the spinal cord almost exclusively through the dorsal root, and synapse in the dorsal horn of the spinal cord, where they project to higher levels such as the thalamus, hypothalamus, reticular system and cortex of the brain (Figure 1.2).

Roughly speaking, the higher-level sites bring about the aversive emotional feelings (thalamus and limbic system), alterations in sleep pattern (reticular system and hypothalamus) and stress responses (hypothalamus) that pain may evoke.

The PNS and CNS do not passively transduce stimuli and convey sensory information. Instead, noxious stimuli trigger biological processes that then amplify or inhibit the noxious signal.

Potentiation. After tissue or nerve damage, peripheral nociceptors become sensitized to noxious stimuli owing to the formation and accumulation of algogenic and inflammatory mediators in the periphery, such as prostanoids, interleukins, bradykinin and histamine. Peripheral sensitization and heightened afferent activity in pain fibers elicit functional, chemical and anatomic reorganization in spinal cord neurons. These changes lead to long-term central potentiation, a form of pain memory characterized by progressively enhanced and prolonged spinal neuronal responses to afferent impulses.

This spatially and temporally exaggerated processing of persistent nociceptive information translates clinically into increased experience

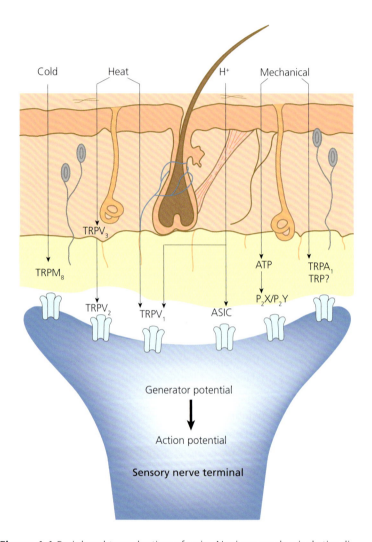

Figure 1.1 Peripheral transduction of pain. Noxious mechanical stimuli release ATP, which may act on one or more purine receptors (P_2X and P_2Y). A second mechanism may involve transient receptor potential (TRP)A_1 or other TRP receptors. Noxious chemical stimuli such as acidity (H^+) act via acid-sensing ion channels (ASICs) or TRP vanilloid (TRPV)$_1$ receptors. Noxious heat acts via TRPV$_1$ and TRPV$_2$, possibly via TRPV$_3$ receptors. Noxious cold acts via TRP melastatin (TRPM)$_8$ receptors. Adapted from Marchand F, Perretti M, McMahon SB. *Nat Rev Neurosci* 2005;6:521–32 and Wrigley PJ, Jeong H-J, Vaughan CW. *Br J Pharmacol* 2009;157:371–80.

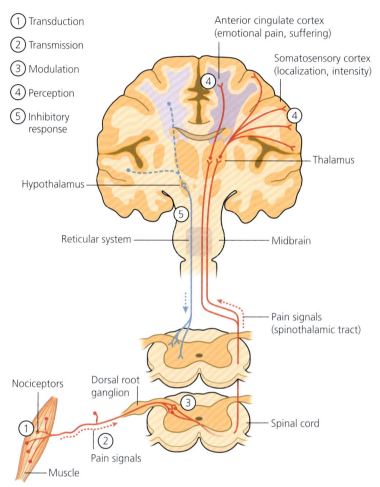

Figure 1.2 Nociceptive pathways. (1) Transduction: conversion of a noxious stimulus into electrical energy by a peripheral nociceptor (see Figure 1.1). (2) Transmission: propagation of the signal through the peripheral nervous system via first-order neurons. (3) Modulation: adjustment of pain intensity at the point where first-order neurons synapse with second-order neurons in the dorsal horn of the spinal cord. (4) Perception: the cerebral cortical response to nociceptive signals projected to the brain by third-order neurons. (5) Inhibitory response: stimulation of the descending pathway from the brain (blue arrow) sends inhibitory responses back to the periphery – the brain can order the release of chemicals with an analgesic effect that may reduce or even abolish some forms of pain.

of pain – not only response to noxious stimulation in the injured tissue (primary hyperalgesia), but also response in the surrounding uninjured tissue (secondary hyperalgesia), with repetitive stimulation producing progressively greater neuronal responses.

Central potentiation is due to the release by spinal afferent nociceptive neurons of excitatory mediators such as substance P and glutamate that bind to neurokinin-1 (NK1) and N-methyl D-aspartate (NMDA) receptors, respectively, in the dorsal horn. Concurrent activation of these receptors allows a massive influx of calcium into second-order neurons, the cell bodies of which lie within the dorsal horn of the spinal cord. Consequently, calcium-dependent intracellular enzymes such as protein kinase C (PKC) are activated, catalyzing the production of nitric oxide (NO) and prostaglandins. These protein kinases also activate other proteins such as ion channels and enzymes (Figure 1.3).

Inhibition. Pain also triggers processes that dampen the perception of nociceptive stimuli. Nociceptive afferent traffic ascends to the midbrain and brainstem, where it activates descending pathways that inhibit spinal pain transmission (see Figure 1.2). These descending inhibitory systems are stimulated by endogenous opioids, as well as monoamines such as norepinephrine (noradrenaline) and serotonin. They inhibit spinal nociceptive transmission through the local release of inhibitory transmitters such as γ-aminobutyric acid (GABA), glycine, adenosine and endogenous opioids at the spinal level.

Analgesics such as opioids, tricyclic antidepressants and serotonin–norepinephrine-reuptake inhibitors (SNRIs), in addition to their other mechanisms of action, activate these inhibitory systems. Furthermore, pain elicits a stress hormone response that includes the systemic secretion of endogenous opioids from the anterior pituitary and the adrenal medulla.

Interpretation
Pain is more than the nociceptive cascade described above. Pain is 'an unpleasant sensory and emotional experience associated with actual or potential tissue damage, or described in terms of such damage' (International Association for the Study of Pain [IASP]).

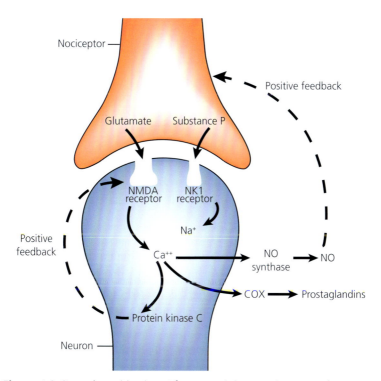

Figure 1.3 Central sensitization. After nerve injury, nociceptors release excitatory mediators such as substance P and glutamate, which bind to neurokinin-1 (NK1) and N-methyl D-aspartate (NMDA) receptors, respectively, in the dorsal horn. This results in an increase in intracellular calcium concentration and subsequent intracellular activation of the calcium-dependent enzyme protein kinase C (PKC). PKC catalyzes the production of nitric oxide (NO). NO and PKC enhance postsynaptic neuronal excitability by increasing the efficacy of receptor ion channel complexes. The influx of calcium also results in the production of superoxide from mitochondria, with potential cell dysfunction and cell death if intracellular calcium stores are markedly increased for prolonged intervals. Increased intraneuronal calcium also increases prostaglandin release. COX, cyclooxygenase.

Because it is an experience, pain itself cannot be measured directly. Pain, like consciousness itself, is constructed by complex brain processes that are strongly affected by a person's attitudes, beliefs, personality and interpretation of the significance of nociceptive stimuli.

Central to the understanding of clinical pain is the concept that pain may be present without an obvious peripheral source or cause.

Mechanisms of neuropathic pain

Definition. Neuropathic pain is initiated or caused by a primary lesion of the PNS or CNS. Patients often complain not only of spontaneous pain, but also of pain from stimuli that are not normally painful (allodynia). For example, a light touch may be described as painful.

Important types of neuropathic pain and their probable causes are shown in Table 1.2, and are discussed in more detail in subsequent chapters.

Pathophysiology. Several neuropathic pain syndromes share overlapping pathogenic mechanisms. Those pain syndromes that have unique pathogenic mechanisms are discussed in the relevant chapters. Among other classifications, pathogenic mechanisms can be considered as either peripheral or central.

Peripheral nerve injury produces axonal membrane hyperexcitability that leads to spontaneous generation of ectopic impulses. In addition, changes in the chemical environment surrounding the

TABLE 1.2
Types of neuropathic pain and their probable causes

Type	Cause
Trigeminal neuralgia	Compression of trigeminal ganglion or its branches
Postherpetic neuralgia	Shingles
Complex regional pain syndrome	Trauma/infection/surgery/inflammation
Diabetic neuropathy	Persistent hyperglycemia (diabetes)
Toxic neuropathy	Chemotherapy, radiation therapy
Central pain	Trauma to the spinal cord; stroke
Phantom pain	Amputation
Postincisional pain	Surgery

Definitions and mechanisms

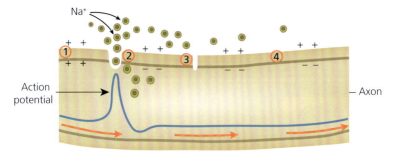

Figure 1.4 Cross-section of an axon with an action potential (AP) moving from left to right. (1) The AP has passed, the sodium channels are inactivated and the membrane is hyperpolarized. (2) As an impulse passes along the axon the membrane becomes depolarized; at the peak of the AP the sodium channels open and Na⁺ ions flow into the axon. (3) Na⁺ ions move in from the adjacent region and depolarize the membrane such that the sodium channels start to open. (4) When the nerve is not transmitting an impulse, a resting potential is maintained across the polarized membrane, with the inside of the axon being negative with respect to the outside.

damaged axon trigger ectopic nerve action potentials, which lead to further impulses (Figure 1.4). Abnormal repetitive firing of injured axons occurs because sodium channels accumulate at the site of injury, creating a lower threshold for the initiation of action potentials (Figure 1.5). Aβ fibers rather than C fibers show the greatest degree of spontaneous ectopic discharge after peripheral nerve injury. Aβ fibers are specialized for light touch and are therefore likely to mediate the allodynia experienced after nerve injury. Nerve injury also triggers the production of a series of inflammatory mediators that promote ectopic activity in primary afferent fibers. These mediators are produced by macrophages that migrate to sites of nerve injury and contribute to chronic inflammation in their immediate environment.

Central effects of peripheral nerve injury. The generation of ectopic impulses is not limited to injured axons; neurons of the dorsal root ganglia with damage to the peripheral axons also exhibit spontaneous activity (Figure 1.6). Also, following nerve injury, sympathetic fibers may sprout and form 'baskets' around dorsal root ganglia cell bodies;

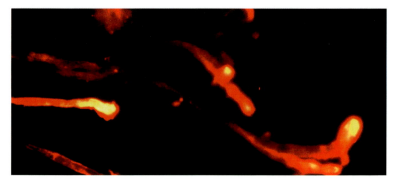

Figure 1.5 Immunofluorescence labeling of sodium channels in a chronic neuroma. The intense labeling (yellow) of the end bulbs indicates an increased density and number of sodium channels. This abnormal concentration of sodium channels leads to abnormally persistent repetitive firing of injured nerves. Photograph provided courtesy of Professor M. Devor (Hebrew University of Jerusalem, Israel).

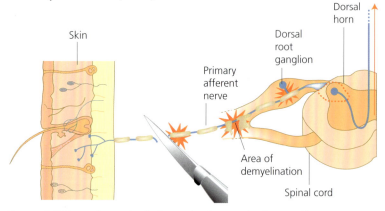

Figure 1.6 Sites of ectopic discharge in damaged primary afferent nociceptors. The regenerating nerve sends out spontaneously active sprouts that are sensitive to mechanical stimuli. A secondary site of hyperactivity develops near the cell body in the dorsal root ganglion (area within dashed line). Ectopic impulses may also arise from a demyelinated section of the primary afferent nociceptor.

at the same time, α_2 receptors are produced on neurons of the dorsal root ganglia. These changes allow for activation of the nociceptive neurons via sympathetic fibers, which themselves are activated by stress.

More centrally, nerve injury activates NMDA and α-amino-3-hydroxy-5-methyl-4-isoxazole propionic acid (AMPA) receptors. This leads to an increase in intracellular calcium concentration and subsequent intracellular activation of PKC and NO synthase, with production of NO. NO and PKC enhance postsynaptic neuronal excitability by increasing the efficacy of receptor ion-channel complexes in the postsynaptic membrane. In addition to the activation of NMDA receptors, spinal cord hyperexcitability could be produced by upregulation of sodium channels and voltage-sensitive calcium channels in neurons of the dorsal root ganglia.

The sensitization (increased excitability) and increased synaptic efficacy of second-order neurons termed 'wide dynamic range neurons' (i.e. neurons that respond to a range of noxious and non-noxious stimuli) could explain the allodynia that patients experience after nerve injury. The central hyperexcitable state and enlargement of the area in the periphery where stimulation evokes a neuronal response are sustained by ectopic peripheral nerve activity that causes ongoing release of neurotransmitters in the spinal cord (see Figure 1.3).

Reorganization of neurons. A variety of neuronal growth factors are released after nerve injury; these can produce long-term modifications in neuronal phenotype and in the structural organization of synaptic connectivity through their ability to potentiate over the long term.

Aβ fibers develop abnormal connections with the nociceptive neurons of the dorsal horn. This structural reorganization may underlie the increased sensitivity to normally innocuous mechanical stimulation after nerve injury (Figure 1.7).

In addition, nerve injury triggers glial activation. Glial cells, the non-neuronal cells in spinal cord and brain, maintain the chemical environment of neurons and deliver the energy to sustain nerve cells. They 'mop up' neurotransmitters released by neurons and release, when necessary, 'glial factors' (the proinflammatory cytokines tumor necrosis factor [TNF]α, interleukin [IL]-1, IL-6 and brain-derived neurotropic factor [BDNF]), which aim to restore balance and aid healing (e.g. in the case of an injured nerve). These substances, both individually and in concert, contribute to the central hyperexcitability by directly activating neurons (Figure 1.8).

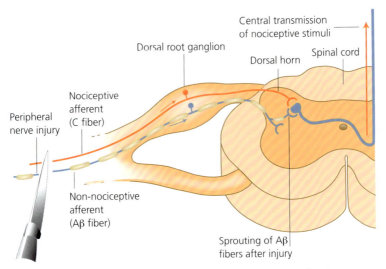

Figure 1.7 Neuronal reorganization and neuropathic pain. Following peripheral nerve injury, persistent pain hypersensitivity may result from new connections between myelinated non-nociceptive Aβ afferent sprouts and nociceptive neurons.

The processes shown in Figure 1.8 can become prolonged, lasting past the time of healing and resulting in chronic neuronal hypersensitivity and persisting (chronic) neuropathic pain. Thus, new treatments for chronic neuropathic pain could focus on the cause of the ongoing pain – overactive glia. At least nine anti-glial drugs are being evaluated. AV411 (or MN-166, ibudilast) inhibits astrocytes. In 2016, it received 'fast track' designation by the FDA for its potential use in multiple sclerosis (MS). Etanercept and the antibiotic minocycline, which both inhibit microglia activation, have shown promise in animal studies but have not proven successful in human studies of pain. The cannabinoid Sativex, which inhibits CB2 cannabinoid spinal receptors on glia, is being studied for neuropathic pain due to MS and in trials of tetrahydrocannabinol:cannabidiol (THC:CBD) extract in patients with intractable cancer-related pain. It has been successful in two of three clinical trials for neuropathic pain in humans. Sativex is approved in many countries for the treatment of spasticity in people with MS.

As glia appear to play a key role in opioid tolerance and withdrawal, these drugs may also slow the development of tolerance to opioids.

Definitions and mechanisms

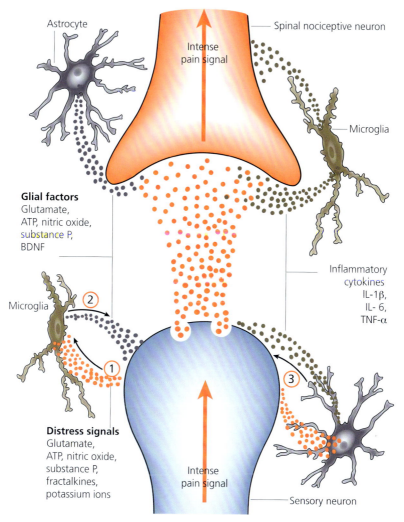

Figure 1.8 (1) After nerve injury, intense signals are transmitted along peripheral sensory neurons to the first synapse in the dorsal horn of the spinal cord. Neurotransmitters cross the synapse to activate spinal neurons. These transmitters are also conveyed to microglia and astrocytes as 'distress signals'. (2) The glial cells produce 'glial factors' and reduce the uptake of neurotransmitters. This either reduces the usual inhibitory processes acting on neurons or stimulates neurons to become hypersensitive. (3) Glial cells are also activated by neural distress signals, which induce the healing process of inflammation through release of inflammatory cytokines, but also result in neuronal sensitization.

Increased glial cell activity normally subsides gradually after injury; its continuation in some patients may be one of the keys to 'what goes wrong in chronic pain'. Chronic use of opioid drugs seems to play a role in glial cell activation, thus increasing pain and decreasing opioid analgesia in a vicious circle (see Figure 1.8).

Loss of inhibition. Moreover, after nerve injury there is also a loss of spinal inhibitory control. Mitochondrial superoxide is produced after the influx of calcium associated with nerve injury, and leads to cell dysfunction and the death of interneurons with inhibitory control. The death of these neurons could explain the decrease in GABA, an inhibitory transmitter, in the dorsal horn of the spinal cord after nerve damage, as shown by immunoreactivity experiments (Figure 1.9).

Finally, the persistent afferent input after peripheral nerve injury provokes changes in the nerve structure of the rostroventromedial

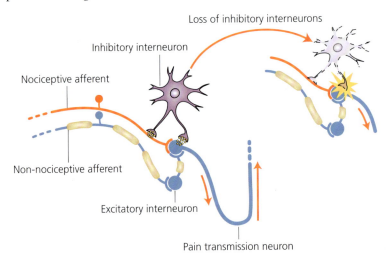

Figure 1.9 Disinhibition and pain. Under normal conditions, inhibitory interneurons actively control sensory inflow. If synthesis of the inhibitory neurotransmitters γ-aminobutyric acid (GABA) and glycine is reduced or the inhibitory interneurons are lost after excessive release of the excitotoxic amino acid glutamate following peripheral nerve injury, the excitability of nociceptive neurons is increased to a level where they begin to respond to normally innocuous inputs. Modified from Scholz & Woolf. *Nat Neurosci* 2002;5:1062–7.

medulla. These changes in turn encourage tonic discharge (firing at regular intervals) of the descending pathways that facilitate nociceptive transmission, further perpetuating the hyperexcitable state observed after nerve injury.

Genetics and pain

Improvements in genetic tools, particularly transgenic knockout mice and microarray-based gene expression profiling, have advanced understanding in this area. In the former, genetic engineering of embryonic stem cell DNA is used to produce a mouse that does not express the target gene. Differences compared with a normal (wild-type) mouse are evaluated: for example, response to different noxious stimuli and to analgesic drugs, revealing six- to tenfold differences in nociceptive and analgesic responses resulting from a single gene manipulation.

In the microarray technique, messenger (m)RNA extracts from tissues of individuals displaying or not displaying nociceptive responses are washed onto a chip that contains DNA probes for thousands of known and unknown genes. Evaluating the degree of mRNA adhesion (hybridization) to the individual DNA probes allows the identification of genes that are expressed differently in the 'pain' versus 'no pain' groups.

Variability in pain response. People report almost ninefold variability in pain intensity in response to a standardized stimulus. This variability is reflected in the degree of activation of 'pain' areas of the brain, such as the anterior cingulate gyrus and somatosensory area 1.

This variation in pain response is reflected in a groundbreaking study of patients with sciatica, in whom a key enzyme (GTP cyclohydrolase 1 [GCH1]) was found to be activated, in turn increasing release of the transmitter NO. The marked individual variation in GCH1 activity and NO release correlated with the pain intensity experienced and the risk of developing persistent pain. Identification of a small family of genes that controls the activation of GCH1 and NO release means that it may be possible to develop a genetic marker, based on DNA testing, to determine which patients are at risk of progressing from acute to persistent pain after injury or surgery.

Specific single gene-related abnormalities in pain experience have been identified in humans. Genetic links have been reported for a number of conditions, including hereditary sensory neuropathy type II and familial hemiplegic migraine. An even higher level of specificity has been reached with the report of a single (autosomal dominant) gene that controls one of ten sodium channel subtypes, namely $Na_V1.7$. Upregulation of $Na_V1.7$ results in the human condition erythromelalgia – a burning neuropathic pain in the feet associated with red warm feet. Presumably, the development of $Na_V1.7$ blockers will lead to an effective treatment.

Conversely, a surprising discovery is the report of three consanguineous families who exhibited a single (autosomal recessive) gene *SCN9A*, mutations of which caused a loss of function of $Na_V1.7$. Individuals with such mutations had a complete congenital inability to experience pain. These findings challenge previous assumptions of substantial neuroplasticity in human pain experience, as $Na_V1.7$ seems to be an essential non-redundant requirement for nociception in humans. Also, individuals with the $Na_V1.7$ 'channelopathy' have normal sensation (apart from absent nociception) and there is no evidence of neuropathy; they appear to lead normal lives unless they become more likely to attempt dangerous and normally painful feats, such as jumping off a roof. In contrast, the previously identified syndrome of 'congenital insensitivity to pain' is associated with a neuropathy; affected individuals often suffer severe permanent injuries in childhood and may not have normal life expectancy.

It may be of interest in the future to determine whether polymorphisms of *SCN9A* can produce not only the complete inability to experience pain but also interindividual variation in response to a standardized pain stimulus.

Memory and pain

There is strong evidence that learning and memory processes play a key role in determining which patients progress from acute to chronic pain, and continue to experience chronic pain. Such learning processes are accompanied by neuroplasticity changes at multiple levels of the nervous system. Encoding of pain memory is enhanced by circumstantial fear; for example, when injury occurs in highly stressful circumstances such as that associated with post-traumatic stress disorder (PTSD). Extinction (unlearning) plays a key role in keeping neuroplasticity changes in check after nerve injury. However, in patients with chronic neuropathic pain, extinction processes may be impaired. Training the patient to extinguish pain-related memory processes may be a crucial but difficult key to treatment. Such treatment may be via behavioral, pharmacological or neurostimulation techniques, or a combination of these. Innovations in all three of these treatment areas already show promise.

The brain and pain

New sophisticated methods of brain imaging have identified key regions associated with pain and have provided strong evidence that neuroplasticity changes in the brain are associated with chronic pain and accompanying physical dysfunction in humans. A cortical and subcortical network is involved, with the areas most commonly associated being the primary and secondary somatosensory cortices (S_1 and S_2), the anterior cingulate cortex (ACC), the insular cortex (IC), the prefrontal cortex (PFC), the thalamus and, in complex regional pain syndrome, the motor cortex. It is notable that old concepts of a spinothalamic 'pain pathway' provided a very incomplete picture.

The involvement of brain areas of the limbic system (e.g. the ACC and IC) emphasizes the emotional component of the human pain experience and the role that mood and stress comorbidity may have in pain's trajectory toward chronicity and its consequent clinical morbidities. In a landmark study by Coghill et al., the degree of unpleasantness associated with pain stimuli correlated closely with activation of the ACC and S_1. This study provided neural correlates of individual differences in the subjective experience of pain.

Neuroplasticity changes in the brain have been demonstrated in association with postamputation neuropathic pain. Following amputation of an upper limb, the somatosensory cortical area of the brain that once represented that limb is 'taken over' by expansion of the adjacent somatosensory cortical representing only the lip.

In patients who have had a spinal cord injury (SCI), the neuroplastic changes are much greater in those who experience pain than in those with no pain. There is also a correlation between S_1 neuroplastic changes and pain in those who experience pain with the SCI (Figure 1.10). In patients with complex regional pain syndrome, neuroplastic changes in the motor cortex correlate with the motor dysfunction seen in such patients (see Chapter 5).

Neuroplastic brain changes probably parallel learning and memory processes. For example, Akparian and colleagues demonstrated that changes in hippocampal neurogenesis associated with pain-induced mood and stress states affected learning mechanisms involved with the perpetuation of pain. Other mechanisms may include unmasking previously present but inactive synapses; growth of new connections (sprouting), which involves alterations in GABAergic inhibition; and alterations in calcium and sodium channels.

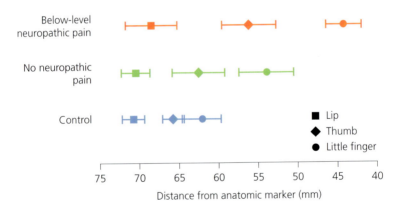

Figure 1.10 Brain neuroplasticity and chronic pain. Distances (in mm) of activated brain regions for lip, thumb and little finger, from a standard brain reference point. Activation by brushing of the skin in the three regions and activation detected in the cortex of the brain (post central gyrus) by functional MRI (fMRI) (mean ± standard error [SE]). Control participants (blue); spinal cord injury (SCI) participants without neuropathic pain (green); SCI participants with neuropathic pain (red).

Pain chronification

The field now recognizes that translation of these mechanisms into a phenomenological trajectory that results in a chronic pain condition is influenced by the confluence of personal, environmental and clinical factors. These factors include genetics, developmental experiences and exposures, previous pain episodes and their outcomes, comorbidities, and treatment factors that increase the risk of acute pain (from injury or surgery or the onset of a disease) progressing to chronic pain and, once pain becomes chronic, progressing to the dysfunction, disability and comorbidities (e.g. depression, substance abuse) associated with chronic pain. This progression of acute to chronic pain and its complications is termed 'chronification' (Figure 1.11).

Every patient requires interventions tailored to change this trajectory or reverse its outcomes. Likewise, to address the public health problem of chronic pain, health systems must be designed to promote the prevention of chronification.

This book sets out the principles of assessment and treatment of different chronic pain conditions with an eye toward successful early interventions that prevent chronification, remediate chronification-related dysfunction and promote functional recovery and quality of life.

Developments in pain management

Novel analgesics. Increased understanding of nociceptive transmission and pain pathophysiology, recognition of heterogeneity among C fibers extending to their production of different molecular transducers, discovery of new receptors such as those for vanilloids or growth factors, and identification of new receptor subtypes have already resulted in preclinical and early clinical testing of novel analgesics. These agents will more specifically target receptor subtypes or ion channels, and promise to be more effective and better tolerated than present therapies. Other novel molecules are designed to interact with multiple receptors simultaneously.

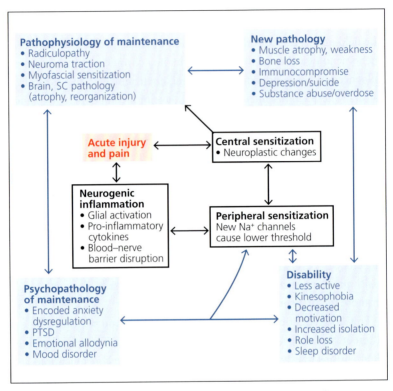

Figure 1.11 Chronification of pain. Following tissue injury, persistent activation of peripheral nociceptors leads to proliferation of sodium channels and glial activation in the spinal cord, initiating peripheral sensitization then central sensitization. Structural changes in the periphery following injury and healing, such as neuroma formation or nerve entrapment in scar tissue after healing, or disease progression such as in arthritis or cancer, perpetuate the peripheral nociceptive stimulus. Anxiety, fear and depression concomitant with pain may further encode pain memory and lower the pain threshold, and the stress-induced increases in pain associated with neuropathic pain conditions facilitate neuroplastic changes in the brain and spinal cord. The disabling effect of prolonged uncontrolled pain leads to new pathology. Each 'stage' in this process must be considered when formulating a biopsychosocial diagnosis and goal-oriented treatment plan in order to control pain in the service of preserving or restoring function and quality of life. PTSD, post-traumatic stress disorder; SC, spinal cord.

Advances in delivery. Setbacks that have followed the introduction of novel agents such as cyclooxygenase (COX)-2 inhibitors have been offset by the development of innovative methods to improve formulations of established compounds.

Iontophoretic or inhalational technology now permits the delivery of lipophilic opioids into the systemic circulation through the skin or lungs. Likewise, intranasal delivery of novel agents (or established agents coadministered with novel excipients) permits more rapid control of breakthrough pain than oral or transbuccal drug delivery.

Advances in imaging technology have taken us beyond a static detailed image of the CNS: we can now see the brain at work. Functional MRI allows real-time clinical observation of the brain's pain excitatory and inhibitory circuitry, which helps us to understand how nociceptive input is processed and translated into pain and suffering. Functional imaging has advanced our knowledge of placebo and analgesic responses, and has even been applied as a novel form of biofeedback to allow patients to control their otherwise refractory chronic pain.

Magnetic resonance spectroscopy appears poised to achieve the Holy Grail of pain assessment: sensitive specific diagnosis of the presence of chronic pain using a quick simple laboratory test.

Pharmacogenetics. No doubt we will be using pharmacogenetics to prescribe analgesics in the future. Each medication will be tailored to the needs and characteristics of the individual, so that each patient will get the most benefit with the fewest side effects. Moreover, pharmacogenetics is already helping us to understand the biological basis for individual variability in response to established agents such as opioids.

Key points – definitions and mechanisms

- The nervous system is dynamic and plastic; noxious stimuli trigger biological processes that lead to amplification or inhibition of the noxious signal.
- Nociceptive input activates descending pathways that inhibit spinal noxious transmission. These descending pathways are potential targets for analgesic drugs.
- Neuropathic pain is produced by a lesion of the peripheral or central nervous system (CNS).
- Nerve injury produces hyperexcitability and spontaneous generation of ectopic impulses in axons and neurons.
- Ectopic peripheral nerve activity contributes to the central hyperexcitable state and enlargement of neuronal receptive fields.
- After nerve injury there may be a loss of spinal inhibition control resulting from loss of neuronal inhibitory processes and persistence of glia-induced neuronal hypersensitivity. The connectivity of sympathetic fibers to injured neurons contributes to the activation of pain by stress. All three of these maladaptions may play a major role in chronic neuropathic pain.
- Increased understanding of chronic pain pathophysiology is leading to new pharmacological targets for treatment.
- Increased understanding of the causal pathway from acute to chronic pain (chronification), provides targets for early preventive interventions following onset of pain-causing injury or disease.
- New imaging (especially of the brain) is increasing knowledge of pathophysiological CNS neuroplasticity changes and showing the effects of biobehavioral training to reverse these changes.

Key references

Apkarian AV, Hashmi JA, Baliki MN. Pain and the brain: specificity and plasticity of the brain in clinical chronic pain. *Pain* 2011;152:s49–s64.

Apkarian AV, Mutso AA, Centeno MV et al. Role of adult hippocampal neurogenesis in persistent pain. *Pain* 2016;157:418–28.

Basbaum AI, Bautista DM, Scherrer G, Lulius D. Cellular and molecular mechanisms of pain. *Cell* 2009;139:267–84.

Binder A, Baron R. In: Cousins et al., 2009 (see Useful resources).

Blyth FM, March LM, Brnabic AJ et al. Chronic pain in Australia: a prevalence study. *Pain* 2001;89:127–34.

Brennan F, Carr DB, Cousins M. Pain management: a fundamental human right. *Anesth Analg* 2007;105:205–21.

Coghill RC, McHaffie JG, Yen YF. Neural correlates of interindividual differences in the subjective experience of pain. *Proc Natl Acad Sci USA* 2003;100:8538–42.

Cox JJ, Reimann F, Nicholas AK et al. An SCN9A channelopathy causes congenital inability to experience pain. *Nature* 2006;444:894–8.

Drenth JP, Waxman SG. Mutations in sodium-channel gene SCN9A cause a spectrum of human genetic pain disorders. *J Clin Invest* 2007;117:3603–9.

Fields RD. New culprits in chronic pain. *Sci Am* 2009;301:50–7.

Fishman SM, Young HM, Arwood EL. Core competencies for pain management: results of an interprofessional consensus summit. *Pain Med* 2013;14:971–81.

Hashmi JA, Baliki MN, Huang L et al. Shape shifting pain: chronification of back pain shifts brain representation from nociceptive to emotional circuits. *Brain* 2013;136:2751–68.

Johnson JR, Burnell-Nugent M, Lossignol D et al. Multicenter, double-blind, randomized, placebo-controlled, parallel-group study of the efficacy, safety, and tolerability of THC:CBD extract and THC extract in patients with intractable cancer-related pain. *J Pain Symptom Manage* 2010;39:167–79.

Melzack R, Wall PD. Pain mechanisms: a new theory. *Science* 1965;150:971–9.

Mogil JS. The genetic mediation of individual differences in sensitivity to pain and its inhibition. *Proc Natl Acad Sci USA* 1999;96:7744–51.

National Pain Strategy (Australia). www.painaustralia.org.au/the-national-pain-strategy/national-pain-strategy.html

Rog DJ, Nurmikko TJ, Friede T, Young CA. Randomized, controlled trial of cannabis-based medicine in central pain in multiple sclerosis. *Neurology* 2005;65:812–19.

Siddall PJ, Cousins MJ. Persistent pain as a disease entity: implications for clinical management. *Anesth Analg* 2004;99:510–20.

Siddall PJ, Cousins MJ. In: Cousins et al., 2009 (see Useful resources).

Wrigley PJ, Press SR, Gustin SM et al. Neuropathic pain and primary somatosensory cortex reorganization following spinal cord injury. *Pain* 2009;141:52–9.

2 Assessment of pain

The initial evaluation of a patient's pain forms the foundation for a rational treatment plan and so it must be as thorough as possible. For patients with chronic pain, this evaluation should include:
- a general medical history, including a detailed pain history
- a physical examination (paying particular attention to neurological and musculoskeletal function)
- a psychosocial assessment
- diagnostic testing (e.g. imaging), when appropriate.

For the busy clinician, a handy mnemonic for assessing the patient's pain history and pattern is PQRSTU (Table 2.1).

Clearly, the history, physical examination and any laboratory evaluation performed to assess chronic pain may overlap with those carried out for general medical diagnosis and therapy.

Many patients with pain due to cancer (see Table 9.1, page 126) or other serious illnesses such as HIV/AIDS experience pain from multiple mechanisms, locations and etiologies. These patients may simultaneously experience: acute and chronic pain; somatic and neuropathic pain related to the primary diagnosis or its treatment; the effects of mood state on pain; or pain from unrelated, possibly pre-existing, common medical conditions affecting the nervous and/or musculoskeletal systems (e.g. neuropathies, spinal pain, arthritis).

Because of the multiple and evolving etiologies of pain, each time a clinician assesses any patient at risk of undertreated pain there must be

TABLE 2.1
Handy mnemonic for the pain interview

P – palliating and precipitating factors	S – severity or intensity
	T – temporal nature
Q – quality	U – you (quality of life)
R – radiating or pattern	

a fresh evaluation of the pain. Unless pain is assessed systematically and classified according to its likely origin as well as its temporal pattern, aggravating and ameliorating factors and perpetuating factors and comorbidities, then the patient is at risk of receiving suboptimal treatment. Even after an initial pain treatment plan is put in place, the source and severity of a person's pain and the effectiveness of treatment may fluctuate, and therefore their pain should be reviewed and documented at regular intervals. The patient is a key partner in this.

History

When taking the patient's pain history, aspects that should be obtained and recorded in detail include: location, duration, type and intensity of the pain; exacerbating or alleviating factors; previous treatments and response to them; and the meaning of the pain to the patient and their family (Table 2.2).

TABLE 2.2
Areas to explore when taking the patient's pain history

- Brief overview of pain site(s)
- History of present illness: include detailed history of current pain and its effects on quality of life and physical and psychosocial functioning
- Past and concurrent medical/surgical history
    - prior patient submission 'time line' (i.e. the chronological sequence of medical and surgical conditions and treatments)
    - highlight significant issues for current pain/treatment
- Family history: highlight chronic pain problems
- Medication (past and present)
    - dose/duration, effectiveness, side effects
    - alcohol, substances, smoking, other
- Other treatments used and health professionals consulted
- Imaging and other investigations
- Psychosocial history
- Review of systems

(CONTINUED)

TABLE 2.2 (CONTINUED)

Detailed current pain history:
- Circumstances associated with pain onset
- Primary site of pain (use of pain diagram; see Figure 2.1)
- Radiation of pain
- Character of pain (using McGill Melzack Multidimensional Pain Inventory [e.g. is pain throbbing, sharp, aching?])
- Intensity of pain (e.g. on visual analog scale)
  - at rest
  - on movement
  - at present
  - during last week
  - highest level
- Factors altering pain
  - what makes pain worse?
  - what makes it better?
- Associated symptoms (e.g. nausea)
- Temporal factors
  - is pain present continuously or otherwise?
  - are there paroxysmal episodes?
- Effect of pain on sleep
- Effect of pain on work and activities of daily living
- Effect of pain on social and recreational activities
- Effect of pain on mood, including anger and anxiety, and if depressed or discouraged, the presence of suicidal ideation
- Expectations of outcome of pain treatment
- Patient's belief concerning the causes of pain
- Reduction in pain required to resume 'reasonable activities'
- Patient's typical coping response for stress or pain
- Family expectations and beliefs about pain, stress and disease
- Ways the patient describes or shows pain
- Patient's knowledge, expectations and preferences for pain management

Adapted from Vije and Ashburn, 2009.

The circumstances surrounding the beginning of the episode should also be documented to ascertain biomechanical and other physical forces that heighten the risk for specific injuries. For example, lifting and twisting causing lower spinal injury, repetitive motion causing tendonitis, a fall from a height causing spinal (or other) fracture or a car accident causing cervical plexus, brachial plexus or traumatic brain injury.

The patient's self-report is a more accurate assessment of pain than vital signs, outward behavior or observer estimates; however, the last is, by default, important in neonates, infants and individuals of any age with severe cognitive impairment or poor language skills. To avoid underestimating pain in individuals with poor cognition or incapable of communicating, indirect indices of pain such as facial expression or body language become more important.

Pain location. It is helpful to ask patients to identify on a body map the areas where they experience pain (Figure 2.1). Body pain maps may help classify pain, as in the case of peripheral neuropathic pain with different causes (see Chapter 6).

Pain radiation. Identification of pain radiation, where present, may be of assistance in evaluating the possible source of pain (e.g. pain from a compressed spinal nerve may radiate down the leg to the foot or down the arm to the hand).

Pain character may help to differentiate somatic, visceral and neuropathic pain. Neuropathic pain can be diagnosed more accurately if a validated instrument is used as illustrated by Table 2.3.

Pain intensity is the most frequently evaluated dimension of pain. During the titration of analgesics for acute time-limited pain of obvious cause (e.g. dental extraction), it may suffice to monitor only pain intensity and forego tracking of other aspects of the multidimensional pain experience.

Assessment tools. Five types of assessment tool have been commonly used to quantify pain intensity (Figures 2.2 and 2.3). The

Patient Name: _____
Date: _____
Clinician Name: _____

1. Indicate (in blue ink) on the figures below area(s) of consistent pain.
2. Indicate (in red ink) on the figures below area(s) of intermittent chronic pain.
3. Indicate level of pain on the scale below.

0   1   2   3   4   5   6   7   8   9   10
no pain   worst imaginable pain

4. Describe how the above indicated pain affects your functioning:
_____
_____
_____

5. Other: _____
Clinician: _____

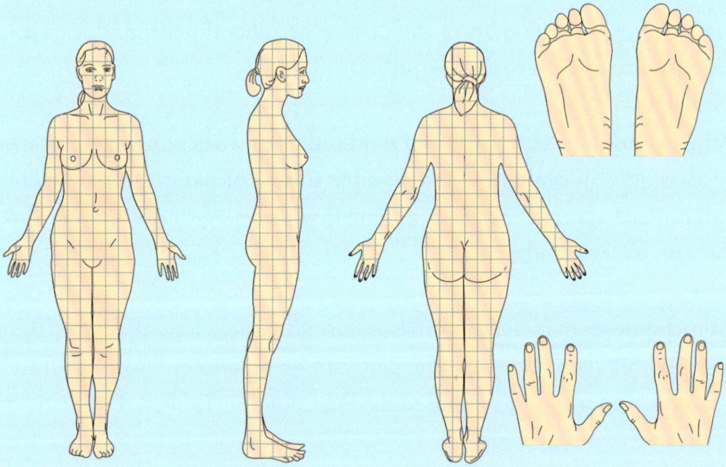

Figure 2.1 Pain assessment form, including a body map, which can be used to document pain symptoms such as location and intensity.

visual analog scale (VAS) is presented graphically with a 10-cm line and endpoint descriptors. Patients place a mark on the line at a point that best represents their pain. Their responses are scored by

TABLE 2.3
Screening tools for neuropathic pain

Items	S-LANSS	painDETECT
Pricking, tingling	+	+
Electric shocks/shooting	+	+
Hot or burning	+	+
Numbness	–	+
Pain evoked by light touch	+	+
Other symptoms	Autonomic changes	Temporal and referred patterns
Clinical examination	Brush allodynia Raised pinprick threshold	Pain evoked by hot/cold stimuli

painDETECT, questionnaire designed to identify neuropathic components in patients with back pain; S-LANSS, self-report version of the Leeds Assessment of Neuropathic Symptoms and Signs pain scale.
Adapted from Bennett et al., *Pain* 2007;127:199–203.

measuring the distance of the mark from the leftmost end of the scale (the 'anchor'). This scale is used primarily in research studies. The numeric rating scale (NRS) may be presented graphically or verbally, with 0 representing 'no pain' and 10 representing 'the worst possible pain'. Patients volunteer a number that best represents their pain intensity. A change of two points on the scale is clinically meaningful. The adjective rating scale (ARS) employs descriptors of pain intensity such as 'none', 'mild', 'moderate' or 'severe'.

Dissatisfaction with the utility of the single-measure NRS and VAS in busy clinical settings has led to efforts to develop other easy-to-use multidimensional screening tools. The pain, enjoyment and general activity (PEG) scale, a three-question tool that assesses pain intensity, mood and effects on function, has been validated for use in primary care (see Figure 2.2).

Clinicians often anchor the numeric scale numbers with adjectives denoting levels of both pain intensity and function, giving the numbers consensual meaning between patient and clinician.

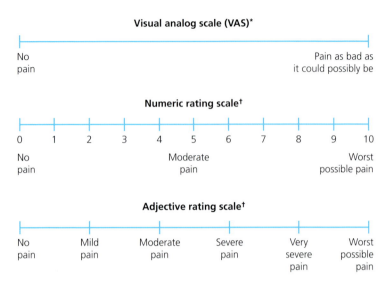
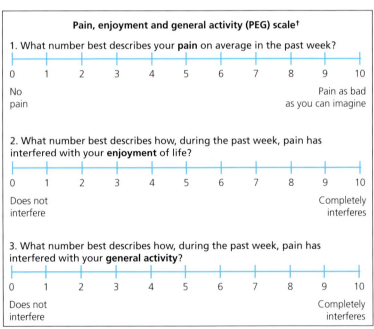

*A 10-cm baseline is recommended for VAS.
†If used as a graphic rating scale, a 10-cm baseline is recommended.

Figure 2.2 Pain intensity screening tools.

Assessment of pain

To standardize use of this clinical advantage (verbal anchors), the Defense and Veterans Pain Rating Scale (DVPRS) was designed for use across clinical settings (including foreign language populations). It anchors numeric pain intensity scores to functional and emotional descriptors, and provides five supplemental questions about common comorbidities (sleep, function, mood, stress) and activity (see Figure 2.3).

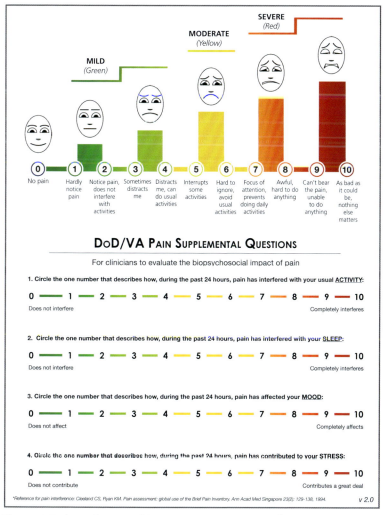

Figure 2.3 The Defense and Veterans Pain Rating Scale (DVPRS), a graphic tool for facilitating self-reported pain from patients.

If these data (or other standardized data) are entered routinely in an online data registry, they can support the clinician's longitudinal monitoring of treatment outcomes as well as clinical research.

Patient's perception. We now know that the decrement in pain intensity experienced by an individual relates to that patient's baseline (pretreatment) pain intensity. The more severe the baseline pain, the greater the decrement in VAS or NRS score needed to achieve clinical importance for the patient.

Examination

It is essential to perform comprehensive neurological and musculoskeletal examinations in addition to other routine physical assessment. The neurological examination should evaluate:
- mental status
- motor system
- sensory perception
- deep tendon reflexes
- cranial nerve function.

Mental status. The items listed in Table 2.4 should be evaluated. The patient may be asked to remember several objects mentioned earlier in the examination, to repeat sentences, to solve simple mathematical problems or to carry out commands of graded complexity. In the case of depressed mood, the clinician should enquire about suicidal ideation, because of the increased risk associated with chronic pain.

TABLE 2.4
Items for assessment in the evaluation of mental status

- Level of alertness
- Degree of orientation with respect to time, place and person
- General appearance
- Behavior and mood (suicidal ideation if depressed)
- Intellectual function, including:
  - comprehension
  - ability to pay attention
  - insight
  - memory

Motor system. An evaluation of the motor system should check the appearance of the muscles (e.g. atrophy), their tone (e.g. flaccid, taut, tender) and strength. Observation of gait can provide information on muscle strength; any indication of impaired vestibular, cerebellar or dorsal column function should be documented. Latent weakness can be detected by asking patients to walk on their toes and heels. Heel walking is the most sensitive bedside test for weakness of foot dorsiflexion, while toe walking is the best way to detect early weakness of foot plantar flexion.

Muscle atrophy can be documented by circumferential measurements of the extremities (e.g. the calf and thigh bilaterally). A difference of 2 cm or more at the same level is indicative of atrophy.

Sensory perception can be evaluated with different types of stimuli, such as light touch, painful squeeze or pinprick (e.g. the sharp corner of an alcohol swab envelope), temperature and pressure/vibration. A freshly opened alcohol wipe may be used as a bedside probe of deficits in cold perception or to elicit cold allodynia.

Deep tendon reflex testing is the most objective part of the neurological examination, as the reflexes are not under voluntary control and testing does not depend on the patient's cooperation. Alterations in reflexes are often early signs of neurological dysfunction.

Pathological reflexes, such as Babinski (foot) and Hoffmann (hand) indicating upper motor neuron dysfunction (e.g. spinal cord compression), should be tested.

Cranial nerve function. The 12 cranial nerves relay messages between the brain and the head and neck. They mediate motor and sensory functions, including vision, smell and movement of the tongue and vocal cords. The evaluation of the fifth cranial nerve (affected in trigeminal neuralgia, see Chapter 4) requires the assessment of facial sensation, jaw strength and movement, and corneal reflexes.

Musculoskeletal examination is important for all patients because of secondary pain related to postural changes, and deconditioning resulting in muscle atrophy, as well as the adoption of abnormal patterns of movement and loss of range of movement in the spine and various joints. All of these can result in a vicious circle of loss of function and increasing pain, as well as a potential for tropic changes. Additionally, certain pain conditions originate in a particular primary musculoskeletal site (e.g. the lumbar spine or other joints). Even in these patients secondary musculoskeletal changes should be sought because of changes in posture, gait and splinting.

Details of what to include in the general and specific examinations are listed in Table 2.5.

TABLE 2.5
Items for inclusion in the physical examination

General examination*
- Observation of posture when sitting, standing, lying and 'at rest'
- Bilateral knee raise
- Squat and rise
- Areas of muscle spasm or trigger points

Specific examination
- All major joints, noting active, passive and resisted range of movement and any local pain on palpation
- Shoulders, particularly, to detect inflammatory or adhesive capsulitis[†] and to examine for brachial plexopathy causing radicular pain down the arm into the hand
- Elbows, for signs of ligamentous or tendonous inflammation
- Wrists, for signs of carpal or ulnar tunnel syndrome
- Hands and fingers for signs of arthritis
- Knees, for signs of abnormal patellar tracking
- Hips, for signs of trochanteric bursitis
- Ankles and feet for postural abnormalities or plantar fasciitis

RED FLAGS IN LOW BACK PAIN (see details in Chapter 10)

(CONTINUED)

TABLE 2.5 (CONTINUED)

Detailed spine examination
- Signs of scoliosis, kyphosis, pelvic tilt
- Palpate midline for tenderness over spinous processes (vertebral bodies) and disks, and paravertebrally for facet tenderness
- Flexion, extension, lateral flexion, rotation
  - pain on flexion may point to muscle spasm
  - pain on extension/rotation or ipsilateral pain on lateral flexion may point to facet-related pain (may also be pain on palpation paravertebrally)
- Sacroiliac joint (SIJ) palpation may be positive in presence of inflammation; various tests of SIJ movement can be helpful
  - straight-leg raising or sitting leg extension that elicits pain radiating to the foot or in the contralateral low back may indicate lumbosacral nerve root irritation or compression from lumbar disk protrusion or spinal stenosis[‡]

Other examinations
- Routinely check blood pressure, pulse, respiratory rate and temperature
- Detailed examination of other body systems depends on patient's history, for example:
  - peripheral vascular system for limb pain
  - thorax and abdomen for abdominal pain
  - abdomen and distal pulses for patients > 50 years with lumbar pain, to check for an abdominal aortic aneurysm

*Should build on any findings from the neurological examination of the motor system. [†]Common with deconditioning. [‡]Often tested in neurological examination.

Psychosocial assessment

The psychosocial assessment should explore the patient's:
- mood, including anger and signs and symptoms of anxiety, depression and sleep disorder – if the patient is depressed, the clinician should investigate suicidal ideation
- coping skills and resiliency
- family and interpersonal support structure
- expectations regarding pain management.

Persistent pain commonly undermines mood, sleep, vitality, function and other dimensions of health-related quality of life (HRQoL). Thus, it is important to monitor how pain and its treatment affect function, daily activities, mood, sleep patterns and other aspects of HRQoL. Scales such as the Brief Pain Inventory, which evaluates pain intensity and the effect of pain on mood, sleep, social function and activities, are commonly used to monitor the effects of treatment from visit to visit.

Quality-of-life questionnaires specifically designed for patients with chronic non-malignant pain have been developed in an effort to better gauge how pain and pain treatments affect HRQoL. For example, the Treatment Outcomes in Pain Survey (TOPS) is a 61-item questionnaire (Table 2.6) that augments the SF-36 Medical Outcomes Study with items originally adapted from the Multidimensional Pain Inventory and the Oswestry Disability Questionnaire. The TOPS is validated in cancer and various chronic pain populations.

Assessment for risk of substance abuse

As noted in Chapter 1, glial activation and other neuroplastic changes in chronic pain underlie a gradual decline in the effectiveness of opioid analgesics (tolerance), leading to dose escalation and reduced duration of analgesic effects. Some patients may become anxious about loss of efficiency and may exhibit symptoms and signs resembling addiction ('pseudo-addiction'). Others may develop aberrant behaviors that suggest a risk for substance use disorder (addiction). Recently, it has been recognized that there is a spectrum of responses that require assessment of 'risk of substance abuse' in each patient using opioids, benzodiazepines or other medications associated with physical dependence and the potential for addiction. This assessment needs to be carried out before starting such medications and at intervals during treatment to determine whether treatment is effective and to monitor the risk for abuse, addiction and overdose.

A number of instruments are now available to assess the level of risk for aberrant medication-related behavior, such as the Screener and Opioid Assessment for Patients in Pain (SOAPP) and the Current Opioid Misuse Measure (COMM); they are available for free online at

TABLE 2.6

Example questions taken from the Treatment Outcomes in Pain Survey

1. The following items concern activities you might perform during a typical day. Does your health now limit you in these activities? If so, by how much?

	Not at all	A little	A lot
Vigorous activities (e.g. running, lifting heavy objects, participating in strenuous sports)			
Moderate activities (e.g. moving a table, pushing a vacuum cleaner, bowling or playing golf)			
Climbing several flights of stairs			
Climbing one flight of stairs			
Bending, kneeling or stooping			
Walking more than a mile			
Walking several blocks			
Walking one block			
Bathing or dressing yourself			
Combing your hair			
Writing			
Talking			

2. During the past 4 weeks, to what extent has your physical health or emotional problems interfered with your normal social activities with family, friends, neighbors or groups?

Not at all Slightly Moderately Quite a bit Extremely

3. How much does your pain get in the way of:

	Not at all	A little	Moderately	Quite a lot	A lot
Enjoying your social activities or hobbies?					
Doing any social activities or hobbies?					
Getting along with your husband/wife/ significant other/family?					
Getting along with friends outside of your family?					
The pleasure you get from being with your family?					
How well you can plan things?					

www.painedu.org. Critical to outcomes is the balance between caution by eliminating or managing risks such as co-prescribed benzodiazepines, depression or substance abuse, and effective management of pain to prevent chronification and its associated pathologies, including overdose by suicide in patients with chronic pain and depression who see no hope for the future. The stratification tool for opioid risk mitigation (STORM) is a new approach to risk assessment for opioid overdose. Statistically derived from a large population sample, STORM is a predictive tool for risk assessment of any individual patient.

Diagnostic tests

Imaging tests can help physicians confirm or rule out diagnoses suggested by findings in the medical history or physical examination. Radiographs provide details of bone structure, while bone scans are performed to rule out occult fractures (small fractures not visible on routine radiographs) or inflammatory processes (such as infection or certain tumors). Bone scans also help determine whether a compression fracture of the vertebral body is old or new, as an old fracture will not 'light up', but a new one will. However, they cannot differentiate between tumor, infection or fracture with adjoining inflammation. In such cases, CT or MRI can better characterize the lesion.

Similarly, in patients whose findings suggest nerve impairment, CT or MRI can help define a possible anatomic cause. However, there is no 1:1 relationship between imaging findings and pain. Indeed, severe degenerative changes may be present with no accompanying pain and vice versa. Imaging studies are therefore no substitute for careful history taking and physical examination.

Key points – assessment of pain

- A thorough evaluation of pain history and a detailed examination are the foundations for a rational treatment plan.
- Persistent pain is a disease entity per se that can undermine many dimensions of health-related quality of life.
- The patient's pain history should document the onset, location, radiation, duration, type (character) and intensity of pain, exacerbating or alleviating factors, previous treatments and response to them, and the meaning of the pain to the patient and their family.
- Assessment of patients with chronic pain should include a physical examination with particular attention to neurological and musculoskeletal function, a psychosocial assessment and, when appropriate, diagnostic testing such as imaging.
- Particular attention must be paid to risks for addiction and/or overdose before prescribing, and during a course of, opioid analgesics.

Key references

Ballantyne JC, LaForge KS. Opioid dependence and addiction during opioid treatment of chronic pain. *Pain* 2007;129:235–55.

Baron R, Maier C, Attal N et al. Peripheral neuropathic pain: a mechanism-related organizing principle based on sensory profiles. *Pain* 2017;158:261–72.

Bennett MI, Attal N, Backonja MM et al. Using screening tools to identify neuropathic pain. *Pain* 2007;127:199–203.

Blyth FM, Macfarlane GJ, Nicholas MK. The contribution of psychosocial factors to the development of chronic pain: the key to better outcomes for patients? *Pain* 2007;129:8–11.

Buckenmaier III C, Galloway KT, Polomano RC et al. Preliminary validation of the Defense and Veterans Pain Rating Scale (DVPRS) in a military population. *Pain Med* 2013;14:110–23.

Butler SF, Budman SH, Fernandez KC et al. Development and validation of the Current Opioid Misuse Measure. *Pain* 2007;130:144–56.

Cheatle M. Depression, chronic pain, and suicide by overdose: on the edge. *Pain Med* 2011;12:S43–8.

Cheatle MD, Barker C. Improving opioid prescription practices and reducing patient risk in the primary care setting. *J Pain Res* 2014;7:301–11.

Cheatle M, Gallagher RM, O'Brien C. Low risk of producing an opioid use disorder in primary care by prescribing opioids to prescreened patients with chronic noncancer pain. *Pain Med* 2017; 31 March [Epub ahead of print] doi: 10.1093/pm/pnx032.

Finkelman MD, Kulich RJ, Zacharoff KL et al. Shortening the Screener and Opioid Assessment for Patients with Pain-Revised (SOAPP-R): a proof-of-principle study for customized computer-based testing. *Pain Med* 2015;16:2344–56.

Krebs EE, Lorenz KA, Bair MJ et al. Development and initial validation of the PEG, a 3-item scale assessing pain intensity and interference. *J Gen Intern Med* 2009;24:733–8.

Nassif TH, Hull A, Holliday SB et al. Concurrent validity of the Defense and Veterans Pain Rating Scale in VA outpatients. *Pain Med* 2015;16:2152–61.

Oliva EM, Bowe T, Tavakoli S et al. Development and applications of the Veterans Health Administration's Stratification Tool for Opioid Risk Mitigation (STORM) to improve opioid safety and prevent overdose and suicide. *Psychol Serv* 2017;14:34–49.

PainEDU. Opioid risk management. SOAPP® and COMM™ tools. www.painedu.org/soapp.asp, last accessed 30 May 2017.

Passik SD, Kirsh KL, Casper D. Addiction-related assessment tools and pain management: instruments for screening, treatment planning, and monitoring compliance. *Pain Med* 2008;9(suppl 2):S145–S66.

Peppin JF, Passik SD, Couto JE et al. Recommendations for urine drug monitoring as a component of opioid therapy in the treatment of chronic pain. *Pain Med* 2012;13:886–96.

Rogers WH, Wittink HM, Ashburn MA et al. Using the "TOPS," an outcomes instrument for multidisciplinary outpatient pain treatment. *Pain Med* 2000;1:55–67.

Trafton J, Martine S, Michel M et al. Evaluation of the acceptability and usability of a decision support system to encourage safe and effective use of opioid therapy for chronic, noncancer pain by primary care providers. *Pain Med* 2010;11:575–85.

Treede R, Rief W, Barke A et al. A classification of chronic pain for ICD-11. *Pain* 2015;156:1003–7.

Turk DC, Dworkin RH, Burke LB et al. Developing patient-reported outcome measures for pain clinical trials: IMMPACT recommendations. *Pain* 2006;125:208–15.

3 Treatment options

Pain chronification and interdisciplinary stepped care

The International Association for the Study of Pain (IASP), the American Academy of Pain Medicine, the Faculty of Pain Medicine of the Australian and New Zealand College of Anaesthetists and the American College of Rheumatology, among many other professional organizations, have long advocated a multidisciplinary stepped care approach that addresses the multidimensional phenomenology of pain chronification (see page 25) as the preferred method of restoring health-related quality of life and functionality to patients with chronic pain.

The high prevalence of chronic pain in the general population and the relatively small number of pain specialists dictates that prevention of chronification largely rests with primary care physicians and clinical specialty teams who are most often present after the onset of pain. Others in the health system, such as surgeons and acute pain subspecialists/anesthesiologists, may intervene effectively with surgical and anesthetic techniques to reduce the incidence or severity of pain chronification after injury or surgery and to identify factors that may influence progression to chronification. Regardless of the setting, patients should be aligned with a healthcare team that has the requisite competencies to evaluate and treat their pain successfully. Partnership between the primary care clinical team and patient, supported by ready access to consultation, and collaborative care with pain medicine and other specialists, enables cost-effective selective use of healthcare resources.

The stepped care model. Using the stepped care model, pain treatment modalities can be added and intensity of treatment increased according to the need to manage factors such as complexity, risks, comorbidities and treatment refractoriness (Figure 3.1). For most patients, attention to all the potential physical, psychosocial, medical, vocational and social aspects of their chronic pain is not necessary, but rather selective

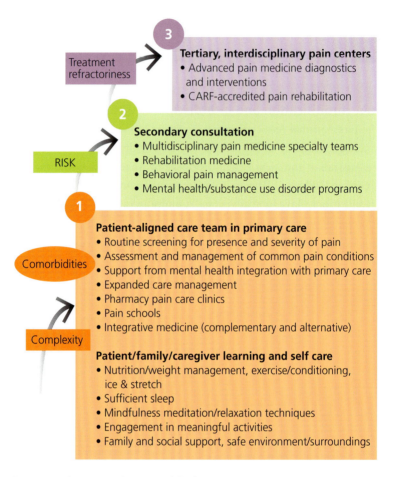

Figure 3.1 The stepped care model of pain management.
CARF, Commission on Accreditation of Rehabilitation Services (USA).

attention is given to the most salient features of their pain condition. Thus, several large health systems in the USA, Australia and Europe have instituted the stepped care model of pain management that begins with patient education and training in self-management and provides additional pain treatments in a step-wise fashion. The foundation of the stepped care model is an informed patient who understands the nature of their chronic pain and can participate fully with their treatment team in planning and instituting appropriate self-management and biopsychosocial treatment.

Many patients do well with minimal resources; for example, instructions in self-management of an uncomplicated episode of low back pain with simple medical and non-medical interventions such as over-the-counter medications, relaxation training/stress management and physical exercises. Other patients with more complexity or risk such as injuries or comorbid conditions (e.g. anxiety, depression, neuropathic condition) who are refractory to self-management alone, will require additional and more focused care such as condition-focused prescription medication and more formal behavioral and physical therapies. A still smaller group will require formal consultation and collaborative treatment with pain specialists, including procedures, complex pharmacology and more intensive psychological interventions such as cognitive behavioral treatment (CBT). The most complex and treatment-refractory cases may require advanced pain medicine procedures and intensive pain rehabilitation programs to optimize pain control, function and quality of life. Of course, 'two-way' movement of patients to appropriate levels of care may also be carried out.

The critical factor is obtaining an early treatment response to prevent chronification (see Chapter 2) by establishing functional networks that quickly move patients to the right level of care for their needs. Too often patients are inadequately evaluated for risk factors for chronicity and treated with escalating doses of medication that only suppress symptoms, such that they begin to develop psychobiological (e.g. depression, anxiety, sleep), physical (e.g. weakness, gait/posture change) and social (e.g. job/family stress and loss) consequences.

Interdisciplinary care. The specific disciplines of healthcare providers needed to offer multidisciplinary care are a function of the variety of patients seen, their complexity and the available resources. The team may include physicians, nurses, psychologists, physical therapists, occupational therapists, vocational counselors, social workers, pharmacists and any other health professional able to contribute to diagnosis and/or treatment.

Treatment is not 'one size fits all'. Ideally, treatment should selectively integrate different modalities following a goal-oriented management plan that is derived from a prioritized problem list based on a biopsychosocial formulation of the predisposing, precipitating and perpetuating factors of the presenting condition. It is crucial that the members of the treatment team communicate with each other on a regular basis, both about specific patients and about overall program development so that treatment is selectively targeted to achieve specific goals. Shared electronic medical records facilitate this process.

Research evidence to support the effectiveness of this approach to chronic pain treatment is just emerging. Meta-analyses of case-controlled cohort studies suggest that, in the case of disability from low back pain, interdisciplinary care increases the rate at which patients return to work and stay at work compared with controls. However, researchers consistently stress the need to improve the number and quality of trials to evaluate the effectiveness of chronic pain treatment programs, particularly the selective integration of two or more treatments to address different pathophysiological pain mechanisms or salient perpetuating factors (e.g. depression). For example, much like the treatment of major depression, a combination of medication and cognitive therapy is superior to either therapy alone, and combining CBT and/or physical therapy with medication and/or injections should be superior to any one treatment; indeed, most clinical experts recommend this approach.

Effectiveness of interdisciplinary treatment. Systematic reviews of the literature suggest that the benefits of interdisciplinary therapy are not uniform across all chronic pain syndromes. For example, for patients with chronic low back pain, cognitive and behavioral treatments such as positive reinforcement of healthy behaviors, modification of patients' understanding of their pain and disability, and graduated progressive physical therapy, all decrease pain intensity and improve functional status. Whereas there is no clinical trial evidence that a similar approach for patients with chronic neuropathic pain syndromes is effective. Nevertheless, most experienced pain clinicians still address stress activation of neuropathic pain with various forms of cognitive-behavioral and relaxation therapies.

The magnitude of the effect of an interdisciplinary approach ranges from slight to moderate. The benefits are less clear when an interdisciplinary approach supplements other standard treatment. For example, behavioral treatment for chronic low back pain has a moderate effect on pain intensity, functional status and behavioral outcomes compared with being on a waiting list or simply receiving no treatment. However, when added to a pharmacotherapy program this positive effect is not observed.

The intensity of the interdisciplinary program also seems relevant. For example, systematic reviews of trials of interdisciplinary therapy for chronic low back pain suggest that although intensive biopsychosocial rehabilitation with a functional restoration approach reduces pain and improves function, less intensive interventions do not produce improvement in any clinically relevant outcome. This may be related to the pathophysiology of chronic pain, in which only intensive biobehavioral training can reverse the central neuroplastic changes associated with disabling pain.

Recent clinical trials indicate that a stepped model of care, with consultative/collaborative care by pain specialty teams (e.g. pain medicine physicians, psychologists, physical therapists) for treatment-resistant or complex cases, is cost effective for patients with low back pain with or without depression in a primary care setting.

Further research. Because of the shortcomings in the methods used in published trials, the cost of multidisciplinary therapy and the increasing need to prove that the cost of proposed treatments is offset by the value they add, more research is needed to demonstrate the benefits of this approach for the treatment of chronic pain.

Active self-management

Rather than resorting to self-help options after pharmacology has failed, active self-management should be the first course of action in the treatment of chronic pain.

Self-management does not mean leaving the patient to their own devices. After appropriate initial education, strategies should be identified to address frequent abnormalities in cognition that lead to behaviors such as fear avoidance behavior, catastrophizing or overdoing.

'Retraining' the brain means reversing the maladaptive sensory and motor neuroplastic changes in the brain that underlie chronic pain.

Although a major aim of self-management is to return the patient to a full range of normal psychosocial activities, the primary care provider and/or other members of the pain team (e.g. psychologist, physiotherapist, as required) must monitor the patient's progress and be alert to the emergence of psychological issues such as anxiety, depression or other issues that may be playing a role in the patient's chronic pain.

Physical activity. There is significant evidence that the motor system can play a positive role in preventing the transition from acute to chronic pain via regular physiotherapist-guided physical activity. Such activity in the motor system helps to wind down sensitization of the central nervous system (CNS). However, patients require 'pacing' strategies in order to avoid 'overdoing'.

Weight management. Clearly, improved quality of life will depend upon improvement in factors within the physical, psychological and environmental domains, which are strongly interactive. It is therefore not surprising that nutrition and behavorial management of weight can play an important role in chronic pain. A poor unbalanced diet can worsen nervous system sensitization, thus increasing pain and undermining attempts to reactivate patients. The weight gain of pain-caused inactivity and depression can worsen disease-caused neuropathy (e.g. diabetes) and joint pain (e.g. arthritis) of the musculoskeletal system.

Relaxation and meditation techniques are also regarded as 'active' strategies, since they can be learned and then applied by patients. Frequent regular use is necessary rather than waiting until there is a severe 'flare-up' of pain. Initial brain imaging studies of meditation reveal the potential for reversing maladaptive brain neuroplasticity changes.

'Passive' management
Although patients may obtain short-term relief from their pain with passive options such as massage or chiropractic manipulation, there

is no long-term reduction in pain. Passive treatments can provide valuable respite in some situations, for example acupuncture for the flare-up of severe migraine, but long-term benefit is rare. Other non-invasive passive treatments include pharmacotherapy (see below), transcutaneous electrical nerve stimulation (TENS) and hot/cold lasers. There are also a number of invasive passive techniques (see below).

A major weakness of all such techniques is that they tend to reinforce the patient's incorrect cognitions, i.e. the belief that the cause of the pain is being treated by a powerful intervention that will fix the problem. Such thinking may steer patients away from more useful 'active self-help' strategies.

Regrettably, some pain management professionals do continue to seek 'the cause' and 'the treatment', while some, who strongly support the use of a broad range of self-help strategies, fail to keep up to date with the risks and benefits of evidence-based 'passive treatments'. Commonsense suggests that a multimodal approach should be used, with a combination of appropriate treatments following a step-wise approach, with the least invasive options given a reasonable trial before the introduction of more invasive treatments, in addition to active self-management. For patients with cancer, major emphasis should be on the cancer itself, as well as some of its treatments (e.g. chemotherapy, radiation, surgery), as a cause of the pain (see Tables 9.1–9.5).

Pharmacotherapy

The pharmacological options for chronic non-cancer pain and cancer pain overlap substantially. However, there are also particular separate issues for chronic cancer pain (as discussed in Chapter 9). Major issues concerning the use of opioids in chronic non-cancer pain overlap, for example, into the 'cancer survivors' group, some of whom may be prescribed opioids over a very long period of time, as can be the case for chronic non-cancer pain.

Multimodal treatment describes the use of a range of treatments, including non-pharmacological and pharmacological options. It can also mean the use of a combination of analgesics acting at different targets. Such an approach aims to optimize pain relief while minimizing the risks of unwanted side effects.

The pharmacotherapy of pain is currently hampered by:
- a lack of drugs with selective action on targets of relevance to pain
- a lack of drugs with reliable potency across a wide population
- marked variation in analgesic efficacy between individual patients (more than sixfold for opioids, and up to tenfold for antidepressants and anticonvulsants)
- no consistency of efficacy for different types of chronic pain, even if the scope is narrowed to neuropathic pain
- a narrow or absent 'therapeutic window' for individual patients and specific analgesic drugs; thus, in some patients effective dose levels cause unacceptable side effects
- a current lack of genotyping for individuals (pharmacogenetics), so that a clinician's only recourse may be titrating different analgesics in successive trials to find one that works for the individual.

In addition, in clinical practice a combination of analgesic drugs with complementary effects are used, whereas most studies compare a single new analgesic with a placebo or existing analgesic.

Opioids

Mechanism of action. Opioid receptors are coupled to ion channels via G proteins. When activated, these receptors modulate calcium and potassium entry into the neuronal membrane. Opioids decrease nociceptive transmission and produce analgesia by hyperpolarizing nociceptive cell membranes, shortening the duration of their action potentials and inhibiting the release of excitatory mediators. However, opioids can also induce a state of increased pain sensitivity (hyperalgesia) even after a relatively short period of exposure. Explanations for this paradoxical effect include prolongation of the neuronal action potential, activation of descending facilitatory pathways, activation of glial cell facilitatory mechanisms, modulation of N-methyl D-aspartate (NMDA) receptors and increased release of dynorphin in the spinal cord. Opioid-induced hyperalgesia may limit the long-term effectiveness of these drugs in some patients with chronic pain.

Efficacy. Many published studies of analgesic drugs only evaluate patients for 12–16 weeks, covering in many cases the duration of acute or subacute pain rather than chronic pain. Although recent opioid treatment guidelines are based on the reality of few if any long-term studies using opioids, a recent review showed that clinical trials of pain treatments rarely extend beyond a few months, partly because of the expense but also because of the ethical problem of maintaining someone in pain when an experimental treatment program is not working.

For chronic non-cancer pain. After a 'tight-fisted' attitude to the use of opioids for both chronic non-cancer and cancer pain, there was a large positive swing toward the use of these drugs in the 1980s for cancer pain and in the 1990s and 2000s for chronic non-cancer pain. Since then, as a result of a rapidly growing death rate due to overdose, there has been another pendulum swing of negative opinion regarding the prescription of opioid drugs for chronic non-cancer pain. This has left some patients with unexpected adverse outcomes and others with a major problem of finding a practitioner who will provide the prescriptions needed to safely and comfortably lower doses or, if appropriate, to wean them off opioids.

Guidelines on use. Defining *which* group of patients with chronic non-cancer pain may benefit from the long-term use of opioids is a challenge. Unsatisfactory initial assessment of patients with chronic non-cancer pain has led, in some cases, to the inappropriate initial prescription of opioids without considering the broad range of potentially more suitable options or the risks for misuse, abuse, addiction and overdose. Illegal diversion of opioid prescriptions for profitable sale as substances for abuse is also a significant problem in the USA.

There is clear evidence that certain factors increase the risk of unintentional overdose. These include concurrent use of sedatives such as benzodiazepines and alcohol, higher opioid doses (> 100 mg morphine) and medical comorbidities such as chronic lung disease. Intentional overdose in suicide, or overdoses associated with misuse in patients with substance use disorders can occur with any prescribed level of opioid dose, and often occurs with other medications too.

Clinical practice guidelines, such as those published by the US Departments of Veterans Affairs and Defense (www.healthquality.va.gov/guidelines/Pain/cot), provide a detailed discussion of the risks and

principles for safe opioid prescribing in pain management, the tapering of opioids and informed consent. Recommendations include:
- avoiding opioids as a first-line treatment
- evaluating and managing risks in all cases
- stopping opioids when they are not effective and avoiding escalation to higher doses
- considering a taper in patients who are taking more than 80 mg of morphine equivalents per day.

Furthermore, since chronic pain is an independent risk factor for suicide, patients with depression are at risk for an overdose of medication, no matter the opioid dose provided. Unilaterally stopping opioids in such patients without adequate pain control may worsen depression, hopelessness and the risk of suicide.

A step in the right direction is the availability of a combination oral opioid (oxycodone) and oral opioid antagonist (naloxone), which produces unantagonized analgesic effects if given by mouth (naloxone in the gut antagonizes oral oxycodone's effect on the gut but residual naloxone is metabolized in the 'first pass' through the liver). On the other hand, attempts to inject this product results in an acute major antagonism and severe withdrawal symptoms due to immediate antagonism of opioid receptors in the CNS.

Another step in the right direction has been the production of new 'tamper-resistant' formulations of long-acting 'controlled-release' oxycodone. The tablets comprise a matrix formulation with a hydrogelling property, intended to deter crushing and reduce the rapid release of oxycodone upon accidental or intentional misuse. However, despite the intention behind the reformulation, these tablets do not mitigate all forms of misuse and abuse.

For chronic cancer pain. Opioids remain the foundation for management of cancer pain of moderate or severe intensity, especially opioids that are full agonists at the morphine receptor (e.g. morphine, methadone, oxycodone, hydromorphone). Partial µ-opioid agonists like buprenorphine exhibit a ceiling effect for respiratory depression as doses increase. However, in the chronic pain setting, where buprenorphine is commonly utilized, this is of limited clinical relevance, as the current available doses are relatively low.

For patients already on a full opioid agonist regimen, agonist–antagonist opioids such as pentazocine, butorphanol and nalbuphine, should be avoided, as they activate the κ-opioid receptor while simultaneously blocking the μ-opioid receptor, thereby risking precipitation of an opioid abstinence syndrome. In this setting, full opioid agonists at the morphine receptor should be used for additional analgesia, particularly for cancer pain. Alternatively, the partial agonist buprenorphine, which is available as a transdermal patch, has emerged as an option for moderate-to-severe pain. Unlike agonist–antagonists it does not precipitate opioid abstinence syndrome, rather producing additive analgesic effects when used together with full opioid agonists.

Meperidine should be avoided except in extreme situations in patients with any form of chronic and cancer pain. Prolonged administration leads to accumulation of normeperidine, a toxic metabolite of meperidine with an approximate 20-hour half-life, which causes dysphoria and seizures. It is also very short acting and has a high risk of abuse.

Increasingly, for patients with substance use disorder whose pain requires opioids for control, experts are turning to buprenorphine for safer pain management.

Effect size. Study results have shown that 1 in every 3 individuals taking morphine obtains substantial pain relief.

Adverse effects. Drowsiness, nausea, vomiting, urinary retention and pruritus are frequent side effects of opioids: 1 in every 3 previously opioid-naive individuals develops at least one of these side effects. The risk of respiratory depression when the opioid dose is carefully titrated to decrease chronic or cancer pain is less than 1% in the opioid-naive patient, although it is higher in older individuals, those with chronic lung disease and those who are also using benzodiazepines. The risk of respiratory depression and all other opioid adverse effects – apart from constipation – decreases with chronic opioid administration if doses are not escalated.

Constipation is almost universal during chronic opioid administration, so when chronic opioid therapy is started a prophylactic 'bowel regimen' should also be initiated, comprising a stool softener and a stimulant cathartic. In some countries, oxycodone and the opioid receptor antagonist naloxone are combined in an oral slow-release long-acting preparation. The naloxone has a local action on opioid receptors in the gut, thus preventing or ameliorating constipation.

Route of administration. Oral administration is the route of choice for chronic opioid analgesia because of its convenience, safety, rapid onset and low cost. A systematic review of the literature has shown that the route of administration does not affect the degree of analgesia. Furthermore, controlled-release preparations are not superior to immediate-release forms in terms of pain relief or side effects, but are advantageous in terms of duration of analgesia – particularly at night.

Tolerance. Commonly, the pain-relieving effect of opioids is assumed to decline with repeated administration – that is, tolerance develops, as has been demonstrated in intact laboratory animals. Yet clinical experience indicates that tolerance to opioid analgesia is rarely the sole reason for dose escalation. The need for high doses of opioid from the start of therapy suggests an opioid-resistant pain mechanism (e.g. neuropathic pain). When abrupt dose escalation is needed, a physical reason is usually apparent (i.e. metastasis or local invasion of a nerve plexus). In fact, in animal models of chronic inflammation, opioid analgesia does not decrease to any great extent during chronic exposure. Therefore, there are valid concerns about decisions to withhold opioids in cancer pain or to restrict necessary dose increases. Studies of the role of microglia (see Chapter 1, Figure 1.8) indicate that glial cell activation plays a role in development of opioid tolerance – as well as increasing pain via central sensitization. Thus, the use of glial-blocking drugs may play a future role in ameliorating opioid tolerance.

Opioid rotation. When the dose escalates to a level associated with unsatisfactory side effects and no physical reason is apparent, opioids should be 'rotated' – that is, the dose should be tapered and the opioid discontinued while another one is started. Cross-tolerance is only partial, and rotation enables clearance of metabolites such as morphine-3-glucuronide, a morphine metabolite. If uncleared, these metabolites could antagonize opioid analgesia. Methadone is a good choice for rotation since its analgesic effects are partly due to an action on the NMDA receptor, which has a key role in opioid tolerance. However, since conversion tables are notoriously unreliable with methadone, because of its variable metabolism and interaction with other drugs, to avoid overdose it should only be used by clinicians with appropriate training and experience.

Risk of addiction. Addiction is defined as the compulsive use of a substance that results in physical, psychological and social harm to the user and continued use of the substance despite such harm. The risk of addiction in patients receiving opioids for the first time for medical purposes, such as the treatment of cancer pain, is very low (see also Chapter 2). However, unless detailed assessment of potential risks is carried out before prescribing opioids for chronic non-cancer pain (see Chapter 2), there is a clinically significant risk of addiction.

Addiction is distinct from physical dependence, although the terms are sometimes inaccurately used interchangeably. Physical dependence is a biological phenomenon defined as the development of an abstinence syndrome following abrupt discontinuation of therapy or administration of an antagonist. Physical dependence may occur during chronic administration of many classes of drugs, including opioids, benzodiazepines, barbiturates, alcohol, β-blockers and the $α_2$-agonist clonidine. Physical dependence is of little clinical importance as long as abrupt discontinuation of therapy is avoided. However, patients with addiction problems do develop cancer pain and chronic non-cancer pain and require special management.

Breakthrough pain describes a typically brief episode of pain above a baseline pain intensity that is controlled by a long-acting or by-the-clock opioid. Treatment of breakthrough pain requires the use of rescue medication that offers a rapid onset of action and short duration. This allows patients to obtain prompt relief while avoiding lingering opioid effects once the pain intensity has returned to baseline. Short-acting oral opioids are used for this purpose. More rapid onset of analgesia can be obtained with oral transmucosal fentanyl (fentanyl lozenges), transbuccal fentanyl tablets or transnasal ketamine. Controlled trials have demonstrated the efficacy of these new options.

New opioid options to help overcome the individual differences in response to existing analgesics, in terms of analgesic efficacy and side effects, include tramadol and tapentadol.

Tramadol has weak opioid agonist activity in addition to serotonin–norepinephrine-reuptake inhibitor (SNRI) activity. Higher doses of tramadol (> 400 mg/day) pose a risk for the development of serotonin toxicity syndrome if combined with SNRIs, tricylic antidepressants (TCAs) or, in particular, selective serotonin-reuptake inhibitors (SSRIs), and seizures.

Tapentadol is a centrally acting opioid analgesic (i.e. it binds at the μ-opioid receptor) as well as a noradrenaline-reuptake inhibitor. This dual mechanism of action supports nociceptive and neuropathic (i.e. diabetic neuropathy) pain relief. Although tapentadol has no mechanism for serotonin activity, there are isolated reports of serotonin toxicity syndrome when tapentadol is used concurrently with serotonergic medications such as SSRIs, SNRIs, TCAs, monoamine oxidase inhibitors and triptans.

Opioid tapering should be carried out in all patients who have been identified, by detailed assessment (see Chapter 2), as inappropriate candidates for opioid treatment, those who are no longer benefiting from opioids or patients receiving very high doses. However, tapering should not be commenced until non-opioid treatments have been started, the aim being to have a multimodal non-opioid regimen in place to replace the opioids. Generally, when dealing with high doses, slow tapering over many months, with strong mental health support as needed, works best. Mostly, tapering can be carried out by the patient's primary care provider who, when completing a rapid taper, should see the patient at least weekly, and is therefore in the best position to spot the emergence of opioid withdrawal symptoms (Table 3.1).

Fast tapering is greatly helped by small doses of the sympathetic (α-adrenergic) blocking drug clonidine, starting with 25 μg three times a day and increasing by 25 μg a day after checking orthostatic blood pressure and response to treatment. The opioid dose should be reduced by approximately 10% per week, with dose adjusted on the basis of patient response. If clonidine cannot be used, small additional doses of opioid are an alternative if withdrawal symptoms are too severe.

Opioid rotation, firstly to methadone, can be helpful in patients on very high doses of opioid, since the NMDA action of methadone helps to block withdrawal. However, conversion to methadone should be overseen by experienced physicians because hepatic metabolism varies considerably amongst individuals and can also be affected by

> **TABLE 3.1**
>
> **Opioid withdrawal symptoms**
>
> - Elevated heart rate
> - Raised blood pressure
> - Increased temperature
> - Sweating
> - Pilo-erection
> - Abdominal pain
> - Limb cramps
> - Feeling of extreme anxiety
> - Craving for extra opioid

other medications frequently co-prescribed with opioids, such as antidepressants and anticonvulsants.

Non-steroidal anti-inflammatory drugs

Mechanism of action. Non-steroidal anti-inflammatory drugs (NSAIDs) decrease inflammation by inhibiting the synthesis of peripheral prostaglandins; they are useful primarily in musculoskeletal pain conditions. NSAIDs also have central analgesic properties that are distinguishable from their peripheral anti-inflammatory effects. They inhibit prostaglandin synthesis in the spinal cord, modulate NMDA receptor activity, activate descending inhibitory pain projections and hyperpolarize cell membranes. All of these actions decrease nociceptive transmission and produce analgesia. NSAIDs also affect nuclear transcription factors and ion (K^+) channel function.

Ceiling and dose-sparing effects. NSAIDs exhibit a ceiling effect for analgesia, and therefore should not be administered above the recommended dose range. At higher doses, there is no incremental analgesic benefit and the risk of side effects increases dramatically.

Consensus, reached after an advisory panel was convened to address the issue of cyclooxygenase-2 (COX-2) safety with respect to the cardiac and cerebrovascular side effects of selective COX-2 inhibitors, prompted withdrawal of rofecoxib and valdecoxib. Celecoxib remains on the market. Although this agent has been associated with an increased risk of cardiovascular events in a long-term placebo-controlled trial, chronic use of traditional NSAIDs, with the exception of acetylsalicylic acid (ASA; aspirin), has also been associated with an increased risk of serious cardiovascular events. Patients in need of analgesics for chronic pain should therefore be informed of the risks, and the lowest effective doses should be prescribed for the shortest appropriate duration.

NSAIDs have an opioid-sparing effect, which can be harnessed for the relief of pain of moderate or severe intensity by starting the NSAID before, or at the same time as, an opioid. Clinical consensus is that the combination of an NSAID and an opioid augments pain relief by producing greater analgesia than that achieved with either drug individually. However, the results of meta-analyses question whether this benefit has been demonstrated in clinical trials.

Effect size. Meta-analyses of randomized controlled trials (RCTs) have shown that NSAIDs are effective for the treatment of cancer pain of mild intensity that does not originate from nerve damage. Trial findings have shown that 1 in every 3 individuals using ibuprofen and 1 in every 5 individuals using paracetamol (acetaminophen) obtain substantial pain relief.

Adverse effects. NSAID use is associated with risks of serious gastrointestinal bleeding, impaired renal function, exacerbation of hypertension or worsening of heart failure, and bleeding due to inhibition of platelet aggregation. Older patients have a particularly increased risk of serious gastrointestinal adverse effects after taking NSAIDs. Trials have shown that 1 in every 111 older patients receiving NSAIDs has serious gastrointestinal bleeding that would not have occurred otherwise.

Paracetamol (acetaminophen) is frequently used for chronic musculoskeletal pain, such as that due to osteoarthritis. However, only 20–40% of patients report 50% or more pain relief. Paracetamol in combination with codeine or tramadol seems to provide slightly greater analgesia than paracetamol alone in patients with osteoarthritis, according to double-blind RCTs.

For a healthy adult, the maximum daily dose of paracetamol is 4 g. This equates to 1 g every 6 hours (4 doses of 1 g/day). However, patients with pre-existing liver disease may be at risk of further liver damage if prescribed paracetamol; they may tolerate only three or fewer doses of 1 g/day. Such patients should have regular liver function checks and should avoid alcohol in combination with regular paracetamol.

Bisphosphonates are analogs of pyrophosphates and are powerful inhibitors of bone resorption. Bisphosphonates are useful for the relief of pain due to bone metastases. A systematic review of the literature of RCTs, however, has shown that their effectiveness is only moderate at best, their analgesic effect is not immediate and their use is associated with frequent side effects. Therefore, they should not be considered as first-line therapy. At 4 weeks, 1 in every 11 individuals given bisphosphonates obtains substantial pain relief and 1 in every 16 patients discontinues the therapy because of side effects.

Drugs used for treatment of neuropathic cancer pain. See pages 95–8 and 101–2 for discussion of anticonvulsants, antidepressants, corticosteroids, capsaicin, opioids and lidocaine (lignocaine) patches. Important 'third-line' treatments in cancer pain include low-dose ketamine infusion (150–500 µg/kg/hour) and/or lidocaine infusion (1–1.5 mg/kg/hour), either of which can be given intravenously or subcutaneously.

Drugs used for the treatment of neuropathic non-cancer pain. As discussed in Chapter 6, different drugs in each drug class have been investigated for the treatment of different subtypes of neuropathic pain. Thus, it should not be assumed that a drug that is, for example, effective for diabetic neuropathy will be effective for neuropathic post-spinal cord injury. Nevertheless, there is some evidence of carry-over from one neuropathic pain type to another. This is why each chapter refers to studies of pharmacological management of specific pain types (e.g. post-herpetic neuralgia, diabetic neuropathy, spinal cord injury pain).

Antiepileptics, antidepressants and other drugs useful in the treatment of neuropathic pain are outlined in Tables 3.2 and 3.3.

TABLE 3.2

Antiepileptic and antidepressant drugs for neuropathic pain*

Antiepileptics
- Drugs acting on voltage-gated sodium channels (see text): carbamazepine, lamotrigine
- Drugs acting on α_2 delta subunit of voltage-gated N-calcium channels: gabapentin, pregabalin (oral)
- Drugs acting on GABA system: vigabatrin (no studies, anecdotal reports only), sodium valproate (weak effect)

Antidepressants
- TCAs: amitriptyline, nortriptyline, desipramine
- SSRIs: fluoxetine, paroxetine, sertraline, citalopram, escitalopram[†]
- SNRIs: venlafaxine, desvenlafaxine, duloxetine, milnacipram
- NRIs: reboxetine
- NASSAs: mirtazapine
- Melatonergic agonist antidepressants: agomelatine

Note: irreversible or reversible monoamine oxidase inhibitors are best reserved for psychiatrists treating patients with intractable depression.

*See also Chapter 6.
[†]Clinical trials do not support SSRI efficacy in pain conditions.
GABA, gamma-aminobutyric acid; NASSA, noradrenergic and specific serotonergic antidepressant; NRI, noradrenaline-reuptake inhibitor; SNRI, serotonin–noradrenaline-reuptake inhibitor; SSRI, selective serotonin-reuptake inhibitor; TCA, tricyclic antidepressant.

Antidepressants act as analgesics via a wide range of mechanisms. TCAs and SNRIs are superior to SSRIs. In future, it is likely there will be individualized pharmacotherapy for each patient and for each neuropathic (and other) pain condition. For the time being, success with particular drug types in some but not other pain conditions gives us clues to improving treatment. For example, it is known that trigeminal neuralgia is a unique neuropathic pain condition with paroxysms (or 'lightning bolts') of pain. The paroxysms are directly related to spontaneous action potentials (APs) in trigeminal system neurons (see Chapter 1). As these APs involve the sodium channels, treatment should include sodium channel-blocking drugs of which carbamazepine is one

TABLE 3.3
Other drugs for neuropathic pain

- Drugs working on NMDA receptors: methadone (opioid)μ, ketamine, dextromethorphan, memantine
- Drugs working on GABA receptors: propofol (i.v. only; general anesthetic), baclofen (for trigeminal neuralgia and muscle spasm; also intrathecally for severe muscle spasms, dystonia)
- Other drugs working on the voltage-gated sodium channels: lidocaine (lignocaine) (i.v. and SCI), mexiletine (oral), flecainide (oral)
- Calcium-regulating drugs (for CRPS and bone secondaries): calcitonin (nasal), clodronate (i.v.), alendronate (i.v.)
- Steroids: prednisone (oral), dexamethasone (i.v.)
- α_2-adrenergic blocker: clonidine (mostly to block 'withdrawal' with opioid weaning)

CRPS, complex regional pain syndrome; GABA, gamma-aminobutyric acid; i.v., intravenous; NMDA, *N*-methyl D-aspartate; SCI, subcutaneous infusion.

example. Basic studies reveal that there are nine subtypes of sodium channel and it appears that the $Na_V1.8$ channel is the most effective for neuropathic pain, while having a wide margin of safety before CNS (brain/convulsions) and cardiovascular system (arrhythmogenic or hypotension) adverse effects. Attempts are therefore being made to develop $Na_V1.8$ and other sodium channel subtype blockers.

Invasive procedures
Invasive options broadly consist of neurolytic (e.g. neurolytic celiac plexus block), neurodestructive (e.g. radiofrequency lesioning or neurosurgical anterolateral spinothalamic cordotomy) or neuromodulatory (e.g. intrathecal or epidural drug administration or spinal cord and peripheral nerve neurostimulation) procedures.

Neurolytic celiac plexus block. Visceral pain from upper abdominal viscera is initiated by noxious stimuli, for example due to cancer of the pancreas, transmitted via visceral nociceptive afferents which traverse the largest of the sympathetic plexuses (the celiac plexus) and thence reach the splanchnic nerves, dorsal root ganglia and spinal cord. Neurolytic block can be carried out at the level of the celiac plexus or splanchnic nerves. Both techniques have similar efficacy with 70–94% of patients receiving immediate good relief, which lasts until death in 75% of patients. However, the safety of the procedure relies on thorough knowledge of the anatomy, technique and potential complications (including paraplegia). The procedure is routinely carried out under guidance of fluoroscopy or CT scan.

An advantage of the splanchnic nerve approach is the much smaller volume required, thus permitting the use of 10% phenol mixed with contrast medium in a volume of 2–3 mL on each side – compared with up to 10–25 mL of absolute alcohol on each side for celiac plexus block. This aspect of the two procedures favors splanchnic block as hypotension is less likely (avoidance of lumbar sympathetic block) and paraplegia risk is reduced (smaller volume for spread onto spinal nerve roots and spinal cord). However, splanchnic block requires placement of the needles one spinal segment higher than for celiac block – thus increasing the risk of pneumothorax. Burton et al. have published a detailed evaluation of risks and benefits.

Other neurolytic procedures such as intrathecal alcohol or phenol are now rarely used because of the greater flexibility and lower risk of side effects of intraspinal drug administration.

Neurodestructive neurosurgical procedures are now much less frequently used for pain directly related to cancer because of the availability of intraspinal drug administration (ISDA) and other regional anesthetic techniques. However, it is rare for ISDA to completely relieve cancer pain, whereas anterolateral spinothalamic cordotomy can produce such a result lasting up to a year or more. Cordotomy can be an important option for patients with intrapelvic cancer involving soft tissues and the lumbosacral plexus, as such patients have severe refractory pain and often have a long life expectancy. However, after variable periods of time, pain may develop on the opposite side of the body (mirror image pain) because of an alternative ipsilateral spinothalamic tract. This procedure requires considerable skill and experience and few centers currently have this expertise.

Radiofrequency lesioning. Cancer patients frequently have comorbidities such as back pain due to degenerative spinal disease. Such problems may be amenable to radiofrequency lesioning.

Intraspinal drug administration has emerged as the most frequently used invasive procedure for cancer pain that is unresponsive to multimodal systemic pharmacological treatment and other non-invasive treatments. The efficacy of ISDA has been confirmed in a randomized clinical trial. Many drugs other than opioids are now used for ISDA in an approach termed 'spinal analgesic chemotherapy' to respond to various types, locations and severity of cancer pain.

The most frequently used ISDA system is a percutaneous intrathecal catheter; however, epidural systems can be useful if local anesthesia is to be used for pain that is well localized (e.g. for mesothelioma-related chest wall pain). Fully implanted programmable pumps can be used for patients with a longer-term prognosis.

Ziconotide (SNX-111) in an intrathecal drug that is 1000 times more potent than morphine. It is approved in the USA for morphine-resistant pain.

Neuromodulation. Defined mechanistically, neuromodulation includes simple interventions such as icing and TENS, which presumably activate the spinal cord 'gating' systems described in Chapter 1 and can be used routinely by patients to help with many forms of mild to moderate nociceptive pain. 'Bio-electrics' has emerged as one of the most promising fields in the neurosciences. Neuromodulation has been described by the International Neuromodulation Society as 'Technology that acts directly on nerves. It is the alteration – or modulation – of nerve activity by delivering electrical or pharmaceutical agents directly to a target area'.

The target areas for both electrical and pharmacological applications are nerves and/or the spinal cord and/or brain. The drug delivery component is described above. However, it is likely that electrical and pharmacological applications will be combined in the near future.

Spinal cord stimulation (SCS) is now more than 40 years old, but progress has been slow because of a lack of knowledge of both the neuropathic pain conditions it aims to treat and the mechanisms by which it provides pain relief. Only about 40% of suitable patients respond to SCS with only approximately a 40% reduction in pain.

Recently, the mechanisms by which SCS provides pain relief have been reported and improvements made in the optimization of the technique using a 'closed loop' system that provides continuous and instantaneous adjustment of the SCS. 'Closed loop' spinal neurostimulation is a new concept made possible by direct recording of evoked compound action potentials (ECAPs) in the posterior spinal cords of patients with chronic spinal pain. ECAP recording allows continuous adjustment of SCS, which prevents both understimulation (loss of effective treatment) and overstimulation (adverse effects). The closed loop system is now in the final stages of clinical trials. In addition, high frequency stimulation (10 kHz) and burst stimulation are major advances, reported in large studies to be successful in over 80% of patients, with much larger reductions in pain than previously reported.

Dorsal root ganglion (DRG) stimulation has been reported to be similarly successful, particularly for neuropathic pain affecting a relatively localized number of spinal cord segments. Given these fundamental improvements, it is highly likely that SCS will play a much greater role in chronic and cancer pain treatment in the future.

Peripheral nerve stimulation. The mechanisms of action of peripheral nerve stimulation (PNS) may be similar to SCS; detailed studies are under way. To date, excellent results have been obtained by placing electrodes (the same as for SCS) in proximity to peripheral nerves such as the greater occipital nerve for intractable migraine and for occipital neuralgia. Careful trials of PNS are essential since it is not possible to select suitable patients for PNS by greater occipital nerve block or by any particular clinical characteristics.

Key points – treatment options

- As chronic pain is a multidimensional interdisciplinary biopsychosocial condition, expert consensus and some research recommends a selective, interdisciplinary, mechanism-based approach as the method of choice to restore quality of life and functionality.
- The specific disciplines of healthcare providers required to offer a multidisciplinary approach depend on the variety and complexity of patients seen and the available resources, as outlined in the stepped care model. Most pain care will occur in primary care settings, but ideally with close support from interdisciplinary teams of relevant health practitioners (e.g. psychology, physical therapy, complementary and integrative medicine) including pain medicine and other relevant specialists.
- The education of patients about their pain conditions, enabling their participation in shared decision-making and the development of self-management skills, is now considered a cornerstone of successful pain management, whether it is delivered at home, in primary care or specialty care settings.
- Research evidence to support the effectiveness of the selective, interdisciplinary stepped approach to chronic pain treatment is not yet conclusive; more research is needed to prove its cost-effectiveness in specific pain phenotypes.
- Pharmacotherapy of chronic and cancer pain is mostly multimodal, combining several different drugs that act on different targets. Pharmacotherapy is often combined with other treatment options.
- Opioids play a major role in cancer pain but data for their long-term effectiveness in chronic non-cancer pain are limited.
- There is substantial variation among patients in dose-response and side effects for individual drugs within a drug category. Thus, careful drug titration is required for each individual patient.

Inguinal PNS for post inguinal herniorrhaphy neuropathic pain is also being studied. Results of studies with follow up to at least 1 year are awaited.

Sacral nerve stimulation (SNS) has been used extensively by urologists, urogynecologists and colorectal surgeons for conditions such as urinary retention or incontinence as well as defecation problems. SNS is gradually being used more for pain conditions such as perineal pain, bladder pain ('interstitial cystitis') and pelvic pain (e.g. pudendal canal stenosis). The results for SNS in patients with neuropathic pelvic pain have been mixed, partly because of technical issues such as insecure anchoring of the sacral electrodes, which can prevent optimal stimulation from being maintained; this has now been resolved with a specially designed electrode. The needles used to insert the electrodes have also improved. The favored approach is trans-sacral via sacral foraminae but the sacral hiatus is another option.

Patients with chronic pelvic pain are often in extreme pain that is unresponsive to all treatments. SNS has the potential to transform many such patients' lives.

Key references

Ang DC, Bair MJ, Damush TM et al. Predictors of pain outcomes in patients with chronic musculoskeletal pain co-morbid with depression: results from a randomized controlled trial. *Pain Med* 2010;11:482–91.

Bair MJ, Ang D, Wu J et al. Evaluation of stepped care for chronic pain (ESCAPE) in veterans of the Iraq and Afghanistan conflicts: a randomized clinical trial. *JAMA Intern Med* 2015;175:682–9.

Blyth FM, March LM, Nicholas MK, Cousins MJ. Self-management of chronic pain: a population-based study. *Pain* 2005;113:285–92.

Bowering KJ, O'Connell NE, Tabor A et al. The effects of graded motor imagery and its components on chronic pain: a systematic review and meta-analysis. *J Pain* 2013;14:3–13.

Burch V, Penman D. *Mindfulness for Health: A Practical Guide to Relieving Pain, Reducing Stress and Restoring Wellbeing.* Piatkus, 2013.

Burton AW, Phan PC, Cousins MJ. In: Cousins MJ et al., 2009 (see Useful resources).

Centers for Disease Control and Prevention (CDC). CDC guideline for prescribing opioids for chronic pain — United States, 2016. www.cdc.gov/mmwr/volumes/65/rr/rr6501e1.htm, last accessed 27 March 2017.

Cousins MJ, Brydon L. Unrelieved pain: are we making progress? Shared education for general practitioners and specialists is the best way forward. *Med J Aust* 2014;7:379–80.

Crawford C, Boyd C, Paat CF et al. The impact of massage therapy on function in pain populations – a systematic review and meta-analysis of randomized controlled trials: part I, patients experiencing pain in the general population. *Pain Med* 2016;17:1353–75.

Davies S, Quinter J, Parsons R et al. Preclinic group education sessions reduce waiting times and costs at public pain medicine units. *Pain Med* 2011;12:59–71.

Dubois M, Gallagher RM, Lippe P. Pain Medicine Position Paper. *Pain Med* 2009;10:972–1000.

Finnerup NB, Attal N, Haroutounian S et al. Pharmacotherapy for neuropathic pain in adults: a systematic review and meta-analysis. *Lancet Neurol* 2015;14:162–73.

Gallagher RM. Advancing the pain agenda in the veterans administration. *Anesthesiol Clin* 2016;34:357–78.

Gallagher RM. Pain medicine and primary care: the evolution of a population-based approach to chronic pain as a public health problem. In: Deer TR, Leong MS, Buvanendran A et al., eds. *Comprehensive Treatment of Chronic Pain by Medical, Interventional, and Behavioral Approaches. The American Academy of Pain Medicine Textbook on Patient Management.* New York: Springer, 2013.

Gallagher RM. Treatment planning in pain medicine. Integrating medical, physical, and behavioural therapies. *Med Clin North Am* 1999;83.823–49.

Guzman J, Esmail R, Karjalainen K et al. Multidisciplinary biopsychosocial rehabilitation for chronic low back pain. *Cochrane Database Syst Rev* 2002;1:CD000963.

Institute of Medicine (US) Committee on Advancing Pain Research, Care, and Education. *Relieving Pain in America: A Blueprint for Transforming Prevention, Care, Education, and Research.* Washington (DC): National Academies Press (US), 2011.

Kroenke K, Bair MJ, Damush TM et al. Optimized antidepressant therapy and pain self-management in primary care patients with depression and musculoskeletal pain: a randomized controlled trial. *JAMA* 2009;301:2099–110.

Moseley GL, Herbert RD, Parsons T et al. Intense pain soon after wrist fracture strongly predicts who will develop complex regional pain syndrome: prospective cohort study. *J Pain* 2014;15:16–23

Office of the Army Surgeon General. *Pain Management Task Force Final Report: Providing a Standardized DoD and VHA Vision and Approach to Pain Management to Optimize the Care for Warriors and their Families*, May 2010. www.armymedicine.mil/Documents/Pain-Management-Task-Force.pdf, last accessed 30 May 2017.

Ostelo RW, van Tulder MW, Vlaeyen JW et al. Behavioural treatment for chronic low-back pain. *Cochrane Database Syst Rev* 2005;1:CD002014.

painaustralia. *National Pain Strategy: Pain Management for all Australians*. www.painaustralia.org.au/static/uploads/files/national-pain-strategy-2011-wfrjawttsanq.pdf, last accessed 30 May 2017.

Parker JL, Karantonis DM, Single PS et al. Compound action potentials recorded in the human spinal cord during neurostimulation for pain relief. *Pain* 2012;153:593–601.

Reid MC, Papaleontiou M, Ong A et al. Self-management strategies to reduce pain and improve function among older adults in community settings: a review of the evidence. *Pain Med* 2008;9:409–24.

Siddall PJ, Cousins MJ. Persistent pain as a disease entity: implications for clinical management. *Anesth Analg* 2004;99:510–20.

Siddall P, McCabe R, Murray R. *The Pain Book*. Sydney: Hammond Press, 2013.

Stamer UM, Stuber F. Pharmacogenetics of anesthetic and analgesic agents: CYP2D6 genetic variations. *Anesthesiology* 2005;103:1099; author reply 101.

Swarm RA, Karanikolas M, Rao LK, Cousins MJ. Interventional approaches for chronic pain. In: *Oxford Textbook of Palliative Medicine*, 5th edn. Oxford: Oxford University Press, 2015.

Tayeb BO, Barreiro AE, Bradshaw YS et al. Durations of opioid, nonopioid drug, and behavioral clinical trials for chronic pain: adequate or inadequate? *Pain Med* 2016;17:2036–46.

Upp J, Kent M, Tighe PJ. The evolution and practice of acute pain medicine. *Pain Med* 2013;14:124–44.

US Department of Veterans Affairs. Management of opioid therapy (OT) for chronic pain (2017). VA/DoD Clinical Practice Guidelines. www.healthquality.va.gov/guidelines/Pain/cot, last accessed 30 May 2017.

US Department of Veterans Affairs. *Opioid Safety Initiative Toolkit*. www.va.gov/painmanagement/opioid_safety_initiative_toolkit.asp, last accessed 30 May 2017.

Vachon-Presseau E, Roy M, Martel MO et al. The stress model of chronic pain: evidence from basal cortisol and hippocampal structure and function in humans. *Brain* 2013;136:815–27.

4 Trigeminal neuralgia

Trigeminal neuralgia is an idiopathic paroxysmal recurrent pain in the distribution of one or more branches of the trigeminal (fifth cranial) nerve (Figure 4.1).

Pathophysiology
Pain is usually caused by vascular compression of the trigeminal ganglion or its branches (Figure 4.2), but bony abnormalities or otherwise inapparent multiple sclerosis (MS) can also be associated with trigeminal neuralgia. Although up to 15% of people with MS have trigeminal neuralgia, it is only rarely (0.2%) diagnosed before MS. Rarely, a space-occupying lesion (e.g. tumor) in the cerebellopontine angle can be a cause of trigeminal neuralgia, particularly if there is loss

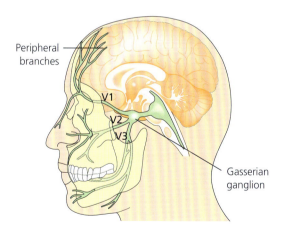

Figure 4.1 Location and structure of the trigeminal nerve. It has three branches (or divisions): the upper first branch (ophthalmic; V1), which runs above the eye, forehead and front of the head; the middle second branch (maxillary; V2), which runs through the cheek, upper jaw, teeth and gums, and side of the nose; and the lower third branch (mandibular; V3), which runs through the lower jaw, teeth and gums. All three branches meet at the Gasserian ganglion.

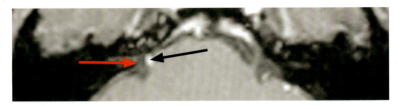

Figure 4.2 Magnetic resonance image showing vascular compression of the trigeminal ganglion in a patient with trigeminal neuralgia. The red arrow points to the right trigeminal nerve (gray area); the black arrow points to the vascular loop (branch of the posteroinferior cerebellar artery; white area).

of sensation in trigeminal territory – sometimes called atypical trigeminal neuralgia. Compression of the peripheral branches of the trigeminal nerve can also occur intraorally or in the region of the chin as the result of trauma, metastatic tumor or injury during alveolar or mandibular bone excision during tooth extraction.

About 5% of people with trigeminal neuralgia have other family members with the disorder, which suggests a possible genetic cause in some cases.

Injury to the nerve root renders axons and axotomized neurons hyperexcitable, particularly in the Gasserian ganglion. A discharge from the Gasserian ganglion is then thought to spread to neighboring neurons, triggering them to fire in turn. Therefore, although trigeminal neuralgia may have an initially inapparent peripheral origin, the clinical syndrome results from abnormal discharges within clusters of central neurons in the trigeminal nucleus and/or abnormal central processing of afferent neural impulses.

Diagnosis

Because there are no objective tests for trigeminal neuralgia, clinical manifestations are the mainstay of diagnosis. Trigeminal neuralgia is more prevalent in women than men by a ratio of 3:2. It can occur at any age, but usually has its onset in individuals over 50 years old.

Clinical features. Trigeminal neuralgia is characterized by paroxysmal and recurrent attacks of facial pain that are sudden and unilateral, and that follow the distribution of one or more divisions of the trigeminal nerve. Pain is precipitated from trigger areas or by innocuous daily activities such as eating, talking, washing the face or brushing the teeth. Patients describe the severe, often excruciating, pain as sharp, stabbing or burning in quality, usually lasting between seconds and less than 2 minutes. A few progress to less intense persistent pain between paroxysms. Remission can be months and even many years, but generally the attacks become shorter over time. Attacks can occur up to 70 times daily, terrifying patients because of their severity and unpredictability despite their brief duration.

Differential diagnosis. Other diagnoses such as idiopathic (atypical) facial pain, muscular pain, dental pain or one of the headache syndromes (e.g. cluster headache or migraine) should be considered if the pain is bilateral or continuous and if there are no evident provoking factors. If there are ocular disturbances, systemic symptoms (e.g. fever, anorexia or weight loss) and tenderness on palpation of the temporal area, temporal arteritis should be considered. Temporal arteritis is a key diagnosis because it can lead to blindness if treatment is delayed. Rarely, a combination of trigeminal neuralgia and cluster headache may occur (cluster tic syndrome) (see Chapter 12).

Imaging. The most important diagnostic imaging technique is MRI. MRI can identify benign or malignant lesions or plaques of MS. In addition, high-resolution MRI (e.g. three-dimensional fast-inflow MRI with steady-state precession) now enables a much more detailed study of the trigeminal nerve and its spatial relation with vascular structures such as a vascular loop (see Figure 4.2). With fast imaging employing steady-state acquisition (FIESTA) sequence MRI, it is important to obtain clear imaging of the cerebello-pontine angle, which is where malignant lesions may occur.

Management
Pharmacological management. Meta-analyses of randomized controlled trials show the anticonvulsant sodium channel blocker carbamazepine, 800–1200 mg/day, to be effective. In general, 1 in 3 individuals receiving carbamazepine will experience pain relief. Frequent adverse events

include sedation, cognitive impairment and dizziness. Rare adverse events are decreased platelet or white blood cell counts and, in the older age group, sodium retention.

Lamotrigine, a sodium channel blocker, slowly titrated to reach 100–400 mg/day, may have an additional effect in patients who obtain insufficient relief with carbamazepine. Other options include the gabapentinoids (gabapentin or pregabalin), particularly in older people or in patients who are unable to tolerate carbamazepine. Pregabalin has an advantage because the dose can be more rapidly titrated than the gabapentin dose, and both gabapentinoids have a lower side effect burden than either carbamazepine or lamotrigine.

In patients with unresponsive pain, it may be necessary to use a systemic infusion of lidocaine (lignocaine), aiming for a blood concentration of 1–2 µg/mL. In adults this usually requires infusion of 50–100 mg/hour (0.5–1.0 mL/hour of 10% lidocaine) delivered via a subcutaneous needle or cannula.

Invasive procedures

If medical management has failed and the patient can tolerate surgery, microvascular decompression of the trigeminal neural complex (also known as the Jannetta procedure) is the preferred treatment. This procedure directly treats the cause of the problem without destroying any neural tissue. Morbidity and mortality are low. Pain relief persists in more than 85% of patients at 5-year follow-up, with no risk of sensory loss. Many patients have complete abolition of pain – a result that is attainable for very few chronic pain conditions.

In older patients, percutaneous radiofrequency lesioning of the affected components of the trigeminal complex is the method of choice. This is a rapid and highly controllable procedure that aims to minimize risk of sensory loss. However, pain tends to recur after about 3 years and about 5% of patients have painful sensory loss (anesthesia dolorosa).

Balloon compression and retro-Gasserian glycerol injection are alternative lesioning procedures. Unfortunately, there are no comparative studies among invasive procedures, so the choice is often guided by operator expertise in a particular technique.

For non-responders and those in whom the pain relief is only temporary, a new or repeat procedure is sometimes performed. The long-term effectiveness of this strategy is unknown, and the risk of producing new neurological deficits is higher. Patients who elect to undergo repeat procedures should be informed of the increased risks.

Because of the severity and unpredictability of episodes of trigeminal neuralgia, patients with ineffective treatment pain are at increased risk of suicide. Risk of suicide is discussed in *Fast Facts: Depression*.

The authors of this text have treated many patients with trigeminal neuralgia who fail to respond to medical management or who have unacceptable side effects. Such patients must be given access to the invasive procedures described above, particularly microvascular decompression (MVD), in view of the high success rate. However, MVD requires a neurosurgeon of high experience in the MVD technique. All neurologists should be knowledgeable about MVD and other invasive options.

Key points – trigeminal neuralgia

- Trigeminal neuralgia is characterized by paroxysmal and recurrent attacks of facial pain that are sudden and unilateral, and follow the distribution of one or more divisions of the trigeminal nerve.
- Pain is usually caused by compression of the trigeminal ganglion or its branches.
- Medical management remains the first line of treatment. Carbamazepine, traditionally the drug of choice, is often replaced by gabapentin and pregabalin because of fewer side effects. Patients hospitalized because of the severity of pain may be effectively controlled by use of a subcutaneous infusion of lidocaine (lignocaine).
- Failed medical treatment is an indication for consideration of microvascular decompression or alternative techniques.

Key references

Devor M, Amir R, Rappaport ZH. Pathophysiology of trigeminal neuralgia: the ignition hypothesis. *Clin J Pain* 2002;18:4–13.

Finnerup NB, Attal N, Haroutounian S et al. Pharmacotherapy for neuropathic pain in adults: a systematic review and meta-analysis. *Lancet Neurol* 2015;14:162–73.

Haddad M, Gunn J. *Fast Facts: Depression*, 3rd edn. Oxford: Health Press Limited, 2011.

Peters G, Nurmikko TJ. Peripheral and gasserian ganglion-level procedures for the treatment of trigeminal neuralgia. *Clin J Pain* 2002;18:28–34.

Rappaport ZH, Devor M. TIC and cranial neuralgias In: Schmidt RF, Willis WD, eds. *Encyclopedia of Pain*. Heidelberg: Springer, 2007: 2482–5.

Sindrup SH, Jensen TS. Pharmacotherapy of trigeminal neuralgia. *Clin J Pain* 2002;18:22–7.

Zakrzewska JM. Diagnosis and differential diagnosis of trigeminal neuralgia. *Clin J Pain* 2002;18: 14–21.

Zakrzewska JM, Linskey ME. Trigeminal neuralgia. *BMJ* 2014;3487:g474.

5 Complex regional pain syndrome

The term 'complex regional pain syndrome' (CRPS) was coined in 1995 by the International Association for the Study of Pain (IASP) to replace terms previously used to describe the condition. The diagnosis of CRPS requires the presence of several factors, which may include sensory, vascular and motor abnormalities as well as edema and sweating abnormalities. The syndrome encompasses an array of painful conditions characterized by continuing (spontaneous and/or evoked) regional pain that is seemingly disproportionate in time or degree to the usual course of any known trauma or other lesion. The pain is regional (that is, not in a specific nerve territory or dermatome) and usually has a distal predominance of abnormal sensory, motor, sudomotor, vasomotor and/or trophic findings. The syndrome shows variable progression over time. Harden et al. have published statistically derived criteria (the 'Budapest criteria') for clinical diagnosis (Table 5.1). More information on diagnosis is also available from the IASP (Table 5.2).

A conservative estimate of the combined incidence of CRPS types I and II is 6 new cases per 100 000 person-years at risk and a prevalence of about 21 per 100 000 people. CRPS type I, previously called 'reflex sympathetic dystrophy', in which there is no definable lesion, develops more often than CRPS type II, previously called 'causalgia', in which there is a defined nerve lesion. The incidence of CRPS II in peripheral nerve injury varies from 2% to 14% in different studies, with a mean of 4%. The incidence of CRPS I is 1–2% after fractures, 12% after brain lesions, 5% after myocardial infarction and 0.7% after total knee replacement surgery.

Pathophysiology

CRPS may be triggered by a variety of events, such as trauma, surgery, inflammatory processes, cerebrovascular accidents and nerve injury. No precipitating factor can be identified in approximately 10% of cases.

TABLE 5.1
'Budapest criteria' for diagnosis of CRPS

The following criteria must be met for a clinical diagnosis:
- Continuing pain, which is disproportionate to any inciting event
- Must report at least one symptom in **three of the four** following categories:
  - sensory: reports of hyperesthesia and/or allodynia
  - vasomotor: reports of temperature asymmetry and/or skin color changes and/or skin color asymmetry
  - sudomotor/edema: reports of edema and/or sweating changes and/or sweating asymmetry
  - motor/trophic: reports of decreased range of motion and/or motor dysfunction (weakness, tremor, dystonia) and/or trophic changes (hair, nail, skin)
- Must display at least **one sign** at the time of evaluation in **two or more** of the following categories
  - sensory: evidence of hyperalgesia (to pinprick) and/or allodynia (to light touch and/or temperature sensation and/or deep somatic pressure and/or joint movement)
  - vasomotor: evidence of temperature asymmetry (> 1°C) and/or skin color changes and/or asymmetry
  - sudomotor/edema: evidence of edema and/or sweating changes and/or sweating asymmetry
  - motor/trophic: evidence of decreased range of motion and/or motor dysfunction (weakness, tremor, dystonia) and/or trophic changes (hair, nail, skin)
- There is no other diagnosis that better explains the signs and symptoms

From Harden et al., 2013.

After some initial controversy, psychological factors are now no longer viewed as etiologic contributors (see 'Psychological processes', page 84). In addition to the pathogenic mechanisms common to all types of neuropathic pain, there are some features that are particularly

TABLE 5.2

Diagnostic criteria for complex regional pain syndrome*

Clinical signs/symptoms
Positive sensory abnormalities
- Spontaneous pain
- Mechanical hyperalgesia
- Thermal hyperalgesia
- Deep somatic hyperalgesia

Vascular abnormalities
- Vasodilation
- Vasoconstriction
- Skin temperature asymmetries†
- Skin color changes†

Edema, sweating abnormalities
- Swelling
- Hyperhidrosis
- Hypohidrosis

Motor/trophic changes
- Motor weakness
- Tremor
- Dystonia
- Coordination deficits
- Nail, hair changes
- Skin atrophy
- Joint stiffness
- Soft tissue changes

Interpretation for clinical use
≥ 1 symptoms from
≥ 3 categories each and
≥ 1 signs of ≥ 2 categories each;
sensitivity 0.85; specificity 0.60

*From the International Association for the Study of Pain (www.iasp-pain.org).
† See Figure 5.1.

characteristic of CRPS. Animal studies have shown that nerve injury is followed by:
- sprouting of noradrenergic axons around sensory neurons at the corresponding dorsal root ganglia
- upregulation of α_2-adrenoreceptors
- an abnormally intense response of injured axons to sympathetic stimulation.

The abnormal innervation and excitation by sympathetic stimulation provide a possible explanation for the abnormal discharges in peripheral nerves that are observed following nerve damage as well as the reactivity of pain to psychological distress.

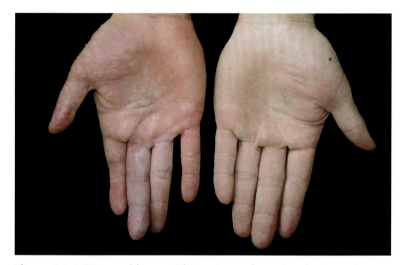

Figure 5.1 A 23-year-old man with type I complex regional pain syndrome. He had a 1-year history of pain in his right hand following direct trauma. He presented with edema and changes in temperature and skin color. The right hand is reddish, with muscle atrophy.

In humans, the nature and extent of involvement of the sympathetic nervous system is less clear (see below). Pain alleviation after sympathetic nerve blockade or sympatholytic drug therapy is not consistent, and relapses are common.

Motor abnormalities, found in 50% of patients with CRPS, are most probably generated by changes in brain motor neurons. Baron's group in Germany has reported disturbed integration of visual and proprioceptive inputs in the posterior parietal cortices of patients with CRPS. Also, functional MRI during finger tapping of the affected limb in patients with CRPS showed reorganization of central motor circuits. The degree of reorganization correlated with the extent of motor dysfunction detected by clinical examination. Thus, it seems clear that maladaptive changes in the brain motor system contribute to motor symptoms in patients with CRPS. This is further evidence of chronic pain as a 'disease entity'. Behavioral/physical treatments aimed at motor components of CRPS in the brain have been described as 'reprogramming the brain'.

Immune-cell-mediated inflammation and cytokine release. Skin biopsies in the affected limbs of patients with CRPS show evidence of ongoing inflammation. Proinflammatory cytokines and high levels of interleukin (IL)-6 and tumor necrosis factor (TNF)α, as well as tryptase (a measure of mast cell activity), occur in the fluid of artificially produced skin blisters. Also, CRPS patients with skin hyperalgesia have been found to have higher levels of soluble TNFα receptor type-1 than patients without hyperalgesia, again indicating a role for peripheral inflammation.

The patchy osteoporosis in advanced CRPS may reflect regional inflammation in deep somatic tissues, as both IL-1 and IL-6 cause proliferation and activation of osteoclasts (bone resorption) and suppress the activity of osteoblasts (bone deposition). There is also some evidence of an autoimmune response in patients with CRPS – possibly triggered by infection with *Campylobacter* species.

However, all of the above peripheral processes do not explain more central phenomena, such as motor abnormalities in the brain, or response to spinal cord stimulation and epidural clonidine (see pages 88 and 89).

Sympathetically maintained pain (SMP) refers to a subset of CRPS patients whose pain is relieved (at least on a temporary basis) by a correctly applied sympatholytic intervention. Those who do not respond are deemed to have sympathetically independent pain (SIP).

Studies in humans by Baron's group now confirm that in both CRPS I and II, cutaneous nociceptors develop catecholamine sensitivity. This appears to occur through a coupling between sympathetic noradrenergic neurons and primary afferent nociceptors at the peripheral level. The actual mechanism of the linkage is different in CRPS I compared with CRPS II. The nerve injury in CRPS II results in coupling at the level of the nerve lesion and also at the dorsal root ganglion. The evidence is less clear for CRPS I. However, it appears that coupling occurs at skin level and in deep somatic tissues.

The pain-relieving effects of sympathetic blocks in patients with SMP outlast the conduction block of sympathetic neurons – in a small number of cases producing permanent relief if applied early in the course of CRPS. It appears that, in SMP, spinal cord sympathetic neurons maintain a positive feedback via sympathetic efferents and then primary afferent nociceptors. Sympathetic block switches off the sympathetic chain, decreases sensitization of afferent nociceptors which, in turn, decreases input to spinal afferents and then to spinal sympathetic neurons. Unfortunately, in most patients, spinal hyperactivity resumes when the block wears off.

The percentage of pain that depends on sympathetic activity declines during the course of CRPS. After about 2 years, there is only a small chance that sympatholytic interventions might be successful.

Psychological processes. There is general agreement that CRPS is associated with emotional and behavioral distress, as might be expected when a person suffers from an extremely painful and often disabling condition with an uncertain prospect for helpful treatment, and often stigmatization. As with most patients with neuropathic pain conditions, psychological distress activates the sympathetic system, and this accounts for the worsening of CRPS pain. There is no evidence of a 'CRPS personality'. The psychological symptoms and psychiatric comorbidities observed in patients with CRPS have a similar distribution in patients with other chronic pain syndromes, supporting the idea that psychological dysfunction is the result of prolonged pain and disability and not the cause of the syndrome itself.

Diagnostic tests

A number of diagnostic tests have been evaluated in patients with CRPS, but diagnosis of the condition remains a clinical one (see Tables 5.1 and 5.2). Radiological abnormalities such as cortical thinning and cortical bone loss (due to increased osteoclastic activity) are often present in CRPS. Patients with CRPS have an abnormal third phase of bone scintigraphy, which is characterized by increased periarticular uptake involving multiple joints in the affected extremity. However, a critical review of bone scintigraphy in the diagnosis of CRPS reported wide variability in scintigraphic changes, with very low sensitivity and specificity. Loss of functional use due to splinting and guarding and changes in regional blood flow could explain the imaging findings.

Treatment

A lack of understanding of pathophysiological abnormalities, and differing views on diagnostic criteria, has hampered the selection of well-defined populations of patients with CRPS to participate in controlled trials of potential treatments. Three literature reviews found little consistent information, and consequently the treatment for CRPS is often based on studies of outcomes from treatment of other neuropathic pain syndromes.

Physical and occupational therapies

Physical therapy, particularly weight bearing, is one of the keys to recovery of function. Particularly in children, physical therapy combined with behavioral strategies can be highly successful. Development of motor imagery using a mirror box and other techniques has proven to be helpful. Such techniques can be described as 'reprogramming the brain', and are aimed particularly at the motor cortex changes now known to occur. Physical therapy and, to a lesser extent, occupational therapy can reduce pain and improve active mobility in CRPS I.

The order of physical therapy strategies appears to be important: laterality recognition, followed by imagining movement, followed by mirror movements.

Psychological therapy

Only one prospective randomized study has evaluated cognitive behavioral treatment (CBT) in children and adults with CRPS, showing a long-lasting reduction in all symptoms in both groups. In the authors' experience, CBT, which helps patients develop coping skills for managing stress in CRPS pain, is a crucial component of treatment and is essential in CRPS of long duration.

Pharmacological management

Non-steroidal anti-inflammatory drugs. There are no studies of non-steroidal anti-inflammatory drugs (NSAIDs) in CRPS. However, from clinical experience NSAIDs help in mild to moderate pain.

Opioids. There are no studies of opioids in CRPS. In the presence of severe pain, opioids should be at least partially effective, as they are effective for other neuropathic pain.

Calcitonin is a hormone produced in the thyroid gland. It has a hypocalcemic effect, inhibiting osteoclastic bone resorption and increasing urinary excretion of calcium and phosphorus. Calcitonin also has a central analgesic effect, but the underlying mechanism is unknown. Naturally occurring porcine calcitonin, synthetic salmon calcitonin and synthetic human calcitonin are all in clinical use. Calcitonin is usually administered by intramuscular or subcutaneous injection, but the intranasal route is also frequently used. Randomized controlled trials (RCTs) to evaluate the benefits of calcitonin in patients with CRPS have shown a small effect at best.

Corticosteroids. Two small single-blind RCTs reported a decrease in pain in patients with acute CRPS after treatment with corticosteroids. The limited sample size of these two studies (n = 23 and n = 36), and the fact that the studies were not double blinded, must be taken into account when considering the significance of the results.

Bisphosphonates. CRPS is associated with increased bone resorption and patchy osteoporosis. Three double-blind RCTs reported that patients treated with alendronate intravenously (7.5 mg/day for 3 days) or orally (40 mg/day) had less pain, tenderness and swelling, and improved motion than those receiving placebo; however, the very small sample sizes (n = 20–32) in these studies preclude any firm conclusion that bisphosphonates are useful therapies.

Tricyclic antidepressants and serotonin–norepinephrine-reuptake inhibitors. Although antidepressants are known to be effective in the treatment of neuropathic pain, only one trial has been conducted in patients with CRPS. Of 48 patients with CRPS type II, those who took clomipramine exhibited greater pain relief than did those who received acetylsalicylic acid (ASA; aspirin).

Anticonvulsants. Although these are effective treatments for neuropathic pain, their use for the treatment of CRPS has not been evaluated, with the exception of one trial that evaluated gabapentin in 307 people with neuropathic pain, 85 of whom had CRPS types I or II. Those who received gabapentin exhibited greater improvement than those who received placebo.

Capsaicin. A meta-analysis of therapies for CRPS and peripheral neuropathy demonstrated that topical application of capsaicin (an alkaloid derived from chili peppers) decreased pain intensity. However, it was difficult to blind the study because of the burning sensation associated with capsaicin treatment.

Intravenous lidocaine (lignocaine) is effective in CRPS I and II in terms of reducing spontaneous evoked pain. In a retrospective case series of patients with severe CRPS who were referred to a tertiary care pain center and were unresponsive to oral pharmacological regimens combined with physical and behavioral strategies, the addition of monitored lidocaine infusions benefited about 40% of cases.

Gamma-aminobutyric acid (GABA) agonists. Intrathecal baclofen effectively relieves the dystonia of CRPS.

Modulation of the sympathetic nervous system. The efficacy of phentolamine and of intravenous regional sympathetic block with guanethidine has not been confirmed in RCTs.

Local anesthetic blockade of the sympathetic chain is a standard clinical therapy for CRPS, but the scarcity of RCTs precludes any conclusion concerning its effectiveness. A qualitative systematic review of observational studies of this therapy suggests that less than one-third of patients treated by local anesthetic sympathetic blockade obtain full pain relief. This rate of success is acceptable to many patients and clinicians, yet its magnitude could be attributed to placebo response, natural history or regression to the mean. Treatment early in the course of CRPS appears to be more effective than in well-established CRPS.

Invasive procedures

Invasive procedures should not be considered in the early treatment of CRPS. Evidence supporting their use is scarce and, to date, only short follow-up periods have been reported. These therapies should, therefore, be offered only in the context of multidisciplinary treatment and after careful screening and patient selection. Nevertheless, the dilemma associated with the use of invasive techniques is that they seem to be more successful when applied early in the course of the condition. Thus, a stepwise approach to non-invasive treatment should be pursued with deliberate speed.

Surgical sympathectomy. Definitive sympathectomy by surgical division, neurolytic nerve blocks or radiofrequency lesioning is not recommended as none provides long-lasting pain relief. In fact, surgical sympathectomy frequently leads to new or worsened chronic pain.

Spinal cord stimulation. In case series of treatments such as peripheral nerve stimulation (PNS) with an implantable programmable generator and spinal cord stimulation (SCS), up to 15% of the systems have to be removed owing to lack of lasting pain relief. The only RCT to date reported that 37% of a small sample of 36 patients achieved substantial improvement in their global assessment but with no improvement in functional status 2 years after treatment started. This study did not employ intensive CBT or other rehabilitation therapies to address functional deficits.

Nevertheless, in severe and refractory cases of CRPS a trial of SCS may be reasonable, particularly if any pain relief is paired with behavioral and physical therapies targeted at improving function and potentially reversing neuroplastic and behavioral changes associated with CRPS. Objective evidence of improvement should first be documented in a temporary trial (e.g. abolition of tremor, improved range of movement, ability to bear weight) before proceeding with the implantation of stimulating electrodes. In some patients with very severe CRPS causing complete limitation of movement of a limb, reversal of this situation occurs within a few hours of starting a trial of SCS. The trial can be continued on an outpatient basis.

Dorsal root ganglion stimulation shows great promise for CRPS in view of its high level of efficacy for pain relief, its ability to target sympathetic and motor affects, and its particular potency in reaching dermatomal areas that are otherwise difficult to reach.

Epidural clonidine. The same judicious approach as described for SCS should be taken with epidural clonidine. Although some case series have reported beneficial effects, there are no rigorous data for patients with CRPS. However, a trial of epidural clonidine may be appropriate for patients with intractable CRPS, and may help the patient start weight bearing and other activity focused on functional restoration.

Preventive strategies

Patients known to have had a previous episode of CRPS, or who are currently suffering from CRPS, are at risk of triggering or exacerbating CRPS if they undergo surgery of the affected limb or suffer trauma to the limb. There are reports that contralateral injuries may also trigger or exacerbate CRPS. Preventive measures should be initiated as soon as possible. Stellate ganglion block before upper limb surgery in patients with a prior history of CRPS reduced the recurrence rate in one study. In a second study, intravenous regional anesthesia with lidocaine (lignocaine) and clonidine was also effective. On theoretical grounds a number of the pharmacotherapeutic options described above may be effective but have not been studied. In the authors' experience, perioperative low-dose ketamine infusion, combined with gabapentin or pregabalin, has proven valuable. Rarely, epidural clonidine is used where there is severe risk of CRPS exacerbation.

Prognosis

The severity of CRPS, rather than its etiology, seems to determine the disease course. Thus, early intervention to reduce the severity of CRPS is vital. In CRPS I, causal fractures have a higher resolution rate (91%) than causal sprain (78%) or other etiology (55%). In CRPS II, more than 60% of patients were unchanged after 1 year of intensive therapy. However, studies of outcome after more than 1 year of treatment with newer techniques are now needed.

Key points – complex regional pain syndrome

- Complex regional pain syndrome (CRPS) involves abnormalities in sensation, motor and sympathetic function, as well as edema and abnormal sweating, with possible trophic changes.
- The involvement of the sympathetic nervous system in CRPS is likely, but detailed mechanisms differ among patients and remain unclear.
- Diagnosis requires the presence of a number of symptoms and signs in the areas of sensory, motor and sympathetic function in the absence of any other condition that might account for the symptoms.
- Intravenous regional sympathetic blockade with guanethidine or systemic phentolamine lack efficacy.
- Local anesthetic blockade of the sympathetic chain is a default clinical treatment for acute CRPS, but the scarcity of data from randomized controlled trials precludes any firm conclusion regarding its effectiveness.
- Sympathectomy by surgical division, chemical neurolysis or radiofrequency lesioning should be avoided.
- Pharmacotherapy largely relies on studies of treatment of other types of neuropathic pain.
- CRPS warrants a cognitive behavioral and rehabilitation treatment program to improve coping and function.
- Severe CRPS may benefit from a trial of spinal cord stimulation or lidocaine (lignocaine) infusions and/or dorsal rate ganglion stimulation.
- New strategies in 'reprogramming the brain' may be able to address the neuroplastic changes that occur with CRPS.

Key references

Baron R, Fields HL, Janig W et al. National Institutes of Health Workshop: reflex sympathetic dystrophy/complex regional pain syndromes – state-of-the-science. *Anesth Analg* 2002;95:1812–16.

Baron R, Janig W. Complex regional pain syndromes—how do we escape the diagnostic trap? *Lancet* 2004;364:1739–41.

Cepeda MS, Carr DB, Lau J. Local anesthetic sympathetic blockade for complex regional pain syndrome. *Cochrane Database Syst Rev* 2005; 4:CD004598.

Compston JE, Rosen CJ. *Fast Facts: Osteoporosis*, 6th edn. Oxford: Health Press Limited, 2009.

Drummond PD. Sensory disturbances in complex regional pain syndrome: clinical observations, autonomic interactions, and possible mechanisms. *Pain Med* 2010;11: 1257–66.

Harden N, Bruehl S, Stanton-Hicks M, Wilson PR. Proposed new diagnostic criteria for complex regional pain syndrome. *Pain Med* 2007;8:326–31.

Harden RN, Oaklander AL, Burton AW et al. Complex regional pain syndrome: practical diagnostic and treatment guidelines, 4th edn. *Pain Med* 2013:180–229.

Iacob E, Hagn E, Emily J et al. Tertiary care clinical experience with intravenous lidocaine infusions for the treatment of chronic pain. *Pain Med* 2017 (In press).

Maihofner C, Baron R, DeCol R et al. The motor system shows adaptive changes in complex regional pain syndrome. *Brain* 2007;130:2671–87.

Moseley GL. Graded motor imagery is effective for long-standing complex regional pain syndrome: a randomised controlled trial. *Pain* 2004;108:192–8.

Perez RS, Kwakkel G, Zuurmond WW, de Lange JJ. Treatment of reflex sympathetic dystrophy (CRPS type 1): a research synthesis of 21 randomized clinical trials. *J Pain Symptom Manage* 2001;21:511–26.

Veldman PH, Reynen HM, Arntz IE, Goris RJ. Signs and symptoms of reflex sympathetic dystrophy: prospective study of 829 patients. *Lancet* 1993;342:1012–16.

Walker SM, Cousins MJ. Complex regional pain syndromes: including "reflex sympathetic dystrophy" and "causalgia". *Anaesth Intensive Care* 1997;25:113–25.

6. Diabetic and postherpetic neuropathic pain

Diabetic neuropathy

Diabetic neuropathy (DN) refers to a group of heterogeneous disorders that affect the autonomic and peripheral nervous systems of approximately 20% of patients with diabetes mellitus. The neuropathy may or may not be painful, though over 45% of individuals who have had diabetes for 25 years will experience painful DN.

Patients report a spectrum of symptoms ranging from mildly disturbing tingling to severe pain that can interfere with sleep and normal activities. Pain may be burning and constant and there may be intermittent electric-shock-like symptoms. Allodynia may be present as well as dysesthesias. The degree of nerve damage does not correlate with pain intensity, and patients can develop insensitive feet without preceding pain or paresthesias. Table 6.1 lists the major types of painful diabetic neuropathy. Small-fiber neuropathy results in loss of ability to feel pressure on the skin of the feet leading to the development of pressure sores, which commonly become infected and painful. All of the other types of neuropathy can be painful.

Pathophysiology. Persistent hyperglycemia is the primary factor responsible for nerve damage. Hyperglycemia increases oxidative stress in nerve cells because of an excess of polyol (sugar alcohol) in the aldose reductase pathway and increases production of diacylglycerol, which subsequently activates protein kinase C.

In 11% of diabetic patients, neurological signs are evident before the diagnosis of diabetes, which suggests that the pathogenic mechanism in some patients is only loosely linked to hyperglycemia. Glycemia-independent theories include autoimmune damage, damage due to hypoxia, and decreased synthesis of nerve-growth factor and neurotrophins.

Damage to peripheral neurons results in spontaneous firing and increased sensitivity of nociceptors (see Chapter 1). Increased input to

TABLE 6.1
Types of painful diabetic neuropathy

Type	Description/symptoms
Acute mononeuropathy	• Normal tendon reflexes • Vascular obstruction • Truncal neuropathy
Autonomic neuropathy	• Silent myocardial infarction • Gastroparesis • Bladder dysfunction • Disturbed neurovascular flow
Compressive neuropathy	• Sensory loss in nerve distribution (e.g. carpal tunnel syndrome)
Large fiber neuropathy	• Motor weakness • Impaired vibration perception
Small fiber neuropathy	• Paresthesias • No motor deficit • Defective heat sensation • Later, progressive hypoalgesia • Risk of foot ulceration
Proximal motor neuropathy	• Pain in thighs • Weakness • Diminished tendon reflexes • Diabetic amyotrophy

the spinal dorsal horn results in central sensitization and increased firing of dorsal horn neurons. The spontaneous firing of peripheral neurons is associated with a change in the distribution of voltage-gated sodium channels, with an altered subtype representation (e.g. of $Na_V1.8$). This offers a future potential for precisely targeted treatment (e.g. $Na_V1.8$ blockers) at the periphery.

Diagnosis of DN rests heavily on a careful medical history. Neuropathy-type pain (burning, shooting) almost always begins in the distal extremities, often symmetrically, since the longest nerves are most vulnerable to damage.

The American Academy of Neurology (AAN) recommends that patients with diabetes and neuropathy should provide a medical history and undergo a neurological examination, as well as a nerve-conduction-velocity study, quantitative sensory testing and quantitative autonomic function testing. The last two tests evaluate the patient's reaction to vibration, light touch, pain and changes in temperature, as well as proprioception and autonomic function. However, these laboratory tests are not necessary to make the diagnosis of DN and to begin the successful treatment of pain.

To allow primary care providers to detect neuropathy in people with diabetes in clinical practice easily, a simple diagnostic tool has been developed and validated – the diabetic neuropathy symptom score. Primary care providers should ask patients about unsteadiness in walking and the presence of pain, paresthesia or numbness. Each symptom adds one point for a maximum possible score of 4. A score of 1 or higher is considered diagnostic for polyneuropathy.

During the physical examination, clinicians can simply, rapidly and reliably screen patients for polyneuropathy using the vibration test. This test comprises the application of a 128-Hz tuning fork to the bony prominence bilaterally situated at the dorsum of the toe just proximal to the nail bed. The patient is then asked to report the perception of both the onset and the subsiding of the sensation of vibration. Testing should be conducted twice on each toe. Peripheral neuropathy is diagnosed if more than half of the responses are incorrect (five incorrect responses or more out of ten tests).

Prevention. Complications of diabetes mellitus (including infections) are more common with poor glycemic control. Randomized controlled trials (RCTs) have shown that maintenance of near-normal blood glucose levels with intensive insulin treatment is the best approach to primary and secondary prevention of late diabetic complications such as DN, the prevalence of which may be reduced by 64%.

Metabolic treatment seems to be a promising approach. Aldose reductase inhibitors suppress the accumulation of alcohol sugars in nerve cells and thus improve conduction velocity; however, the clinical importance of these surrogates is inconclusive.

Pharmacological management. Antidepressants and anticonvulsants are the medications of choice for neuropathic pain, but side effects are common, and particularly troublesome with tricyclic antidepressants (TCAs). Clinical guidelines recommend serotonin–norepinephrine-reuptake inhibitors (SNRIs; duloxetine, venlafaxine, milnacipran), gabapentinoids (gabapentin, pregabalin) or a TCA as a first-line treatment, as medications with these mechanisms are all supported by findings from more than two RCTs.

Given the risks of addiction, overdose and diversion, treatment with long-term opioids, which have also demonstrated efficacy in more than two RCTs, should be considered as a second-line adjuvant option, and only when the risks are evaluated and monitored.

Antidepressants

Mechanism of action. The analgesic benefit of TCAs can be explained by several pharmacological mechanisms: they inhibit the presynaptic uptake of norepinephrine (noradrenaline) and serotonin within nociceptive monoamine pathways and thereby augment analgesia; they interact with opioid receptors; and they block sodium channels, which may account for their analgesic effect in topical creams.

Efficacy. The effectiveness of TCAs for DN has been confirmed in meta-analyses of RCTs. Trial findings have indicated that 1 in 4 individuals given a TCA experiences substantial pain relief (at least 50% relief). However, 1 in 3 individuals develops minor side effects and 1 in 17 stops the medication because of the severity of side effects. The best-studied TCAs are amitriptyline (25–150 mg/day), imipramine and desipramine (desipramine is not licensed in the UK). With fewer side effects, nortriptylene and desipramine are generally preferred, in lower doses than for depression. In older adults, TCAs are used (if at all) with extreme caution, starting at very low doses, because of the increased risk of side effects and toxicity.

Newer antidepressants such as selective serotonin-reuptake inhibitors (SSRIs) are preferable to TCAs for the treatment of depression, but SSRIs do not inhibit the reuptake of both serotonin and norepinephrine, which appears to be necessary for effect against DN. The 'balanced' SNRI class of antidepressants, such as duloxetine, venlafaxine and milnacipran, are generally efficacious in neuropathic pain conditions.

Side effects. The main side effects of TCAs are dry mouth and sedation, both of which are the result of the antimuscarinic activity of the drugs. Low starting doses and careful titration may help to minimize these effects. Orthostatic hypotension, tachycardia, urinary retention and constipation, sometimes associated with TCAs, often pose a problem in the elderly. Because disturbances of cardiac rhythm may be potentiated by TCAs, a baseline electrocardiogram should be taken before therapy is started. For all these reasons, in general, TCAs should be prescribed cautiously in older patients, and started at very low doses. The main side effects of SNRI antidepressants, which are better tolerated than TCAs, are nausea and vomiting and sexual dysfunction; venlafaxine is associated with an increase in blood pressure at higher doses.

Treatment of patients with neuropathic pain and cardiovascular disease should begin with anticonvulsants or antidepressants with SNRI properties, such as duloxetine, milnacipran or venlafaxine, given the increased risk of cardiovascular events associated with the use of TCAs.

Anticonvulsants

Mechanism of action. Many anticonvulsants block voltage-dependent sodium channels and suppress peripherally generated ectopic impulse activity. However, some anticonvulsants such as gabapentin and pregabalin exert their effect through non-sodium-channel mechanisms. They act upon a modulatory site of neuronal calcium channels. Gabapentinoid binding at this site reduces calcium influx at nerve terminals and reduces the release of excitatory neurotransmitters.

Efficacy. The effectiveness of anticonvulsants has been confirmed in meta-analyses of RCTs. As with antidepressants, 1 in 3 individuals given anticonvulsants experiences pain relief. However, 1 in 4 individuals experiences minor adverse effects or severe symptoms that cause them to stop taking the medication.

Carbamazepine, 400–1000 mg/day, is traditionally used for neuropathic pain. Gabapentin, titrated to 1800–3600 mg/day (lower in older patients and those with renal impairment) usually by dosing three times daily, is also widely used for neuropathic pain. Although evidence from RCTs suggests that gabapentin is not superior to carbamazepine in terms of effectiveness or common side effects, the latter can be more severe with carbamazepine. It is not clear if pregabalin is superior to gabapentin, but because pregabalin is dosed twice daily, it is easier to titrate. Trial data show that 1 in 5 individuals given pregabalin, 150–600 mg/day, experiences pain relief.

Side effects. Infrequent cases of Stevens–Johnson syndrome and lymphoid hyperplasia have been reported in patients treated with carbamazepine, but not in those treated with gabapentin or pregabalin.

One in ten individuals taking gabapentin or pregabalin stops taking the medication because of severe adverse events such as dizziness, somnolence or ataxia. The adverse events are dose related: trial data have shown that, with daily doses of 150 mg, only 1 in 39 individuals taking pregabalin discontinues the medication because of adverse events. Perhaps because the clinical picture indicates fewer severe adverse events with gabapentin and pregabalin, clinicians have widely adopted these gabapentinoids as first-line agents for the treatment of neuropathic pain. Pregabalin is now approved specifically for DN in a number of countries.

Opioids are increasingly used for the treatment of refractory neuropathic pain, regardless of etiology, and efficacy has been demonstrated in clinical trials for up to 16 weeks. Of course, careful screening for risks of misuse, abuse and overdose is essential in the long-term use of opioids, as outlined in Chapter 3.

Efficacy. The efficacy of opioids in neuropathic pain is established in RCTs, but their long-term effectiveness and side effects have not been well defined and abuse of prescription drugs is a growing problem, as are unintentional overdoses associated with higher doses or use with sedatives and anxiolytics such as benzodiazepines that also induce respiratory depression.

A meta-analysis of RCTs has shown that tramadol, an analgesic with a dual mechanism of action (i.e. activating both opioid receptors and descending inhibitory pain systems) reduces pain intensity in patients with postherpetic neuralgia and DN at mean doses of 210 mg/day. As with studies that have evaluated traditional opioids, the follow-up periods in the tramadol studies were short. No conclusion can therefore be made as to whether tolerance causes a decline in effectiveness with chronic use, as might be expected for that portion of the drug's effect that is opioid related.

Side effects. Troublesome side effects, such as nausea and vomiting and sedation, are common. Moreover, adverse effects from longer-term exposure, such as hypogonadism, are now documented. Methadone must be used cautiously with slow titration because of its biphasic hepatic metabolism that may be affected by co-medications, such as antidepressants and anticonvulsants, frequently co-prescribed for pain.

Systematic reviews of RCTs have revealed that about 80% of patients receiving opioids experience at least one adverse event. The small number of patients in these trials, and the short duration of follow-up, mean that key concerns regarding tolerance and addiction risk have not yet been answered for subgroups of patients with neuropathic pain.

Postherpetic neuralgia

Postherpetic neuralgia (PHN) is pain that persists after the vesicular rash of acute herpes zoster (shingles) has resolved. Rarely, the condition occurs despite the absence of an obvious rash. The associated pain is usually mild or moderate in intensity, but it may be excruciating. Typically, a single dermatome is involved, but occasionally more than one is affected. Acute herpes zoster is common, developing in up to 20% of people, though PHN is predominantly a disease of older people (see below).

Pathophysiology. Acute herpes zoster results from reactivation of varicella zoster virus (VZV) that has remained latent in neurons of the spinal dorsal root ganglia since an earlier infection, usually childhood chickenpox (in more than 90% of cases). Risk factors for virus activation include older age, malignant disease including lymphoma, stress, and immunosuppression due to drugs or disease.

When reactivated, the virus replicates and spreads outwards to sensory ganglia and afferent peripheral nerves. The virus causes neuronal loss and inflammatory infiltrates in the dorsal root ganglia, nerves and nerve roots. These changes trigger the pathophysiology associated with neuropathic pain (see Chapter 1).

Interestingly, animal studies have suggested that even in the latent phase the presence of the virus may induce abnormalities in afferent nerve function.

Natural history. Advancing age is an important risk factor for developing PHN. After acute herpes zoster infection, 2% of patients under 60 years old develop PHN, but this figure progressively increases to about 50% with advancing age. The apparent severity of PHN reported in RCTs is higher, perhaps reflecting a referral bias. Other risk factors are the severity of the acute zoster lesions and the intensity of the acute pain.

The duration of PHN is highly variable: at least 30% of all individuals with this type of pain will continue to have severe pain 1 year after the onset of herpes zoster.

Diagnosis. PHN is diagnosed on the basis of a history of shingles and the presence of persistent neuropathic pain in the affected dermatome. Symptoms are experienced around the area of skin where the shingles outbreak first occurred. Patients describe a sharp jabbing burning pain or a deep aching pain, with extreme sensitivity to touch and temperature change. They sometimes describe an itching sensation or numbness and, in instances of cranial nerve involvement, their complaint may be considered simply as a headache. PHN often has three distinct types of pain (Table 6.2). Allodynia may result in extreme difficulty wearing clothes and carrying out self-care.

Prevention of PHN is a key strategy as, once developed, PHN is very difficult to treat.

Pediatric VZV vaccination. Prevention starts with pediatric vaccination with VZV, usually around 18 months and then at 10–13 years to prevent infection (ages for vaccination may differ between countries). A range of different pediatric VZV vaccines have been available since 1999, and are funded by governments in some

TABLE 6.2
Types of pain in postherpetic neuralgia

Constant background pain
- Fluctuates in intensity, often burning
- During recovery becomes absent for longer periods before diminishing in intensity

Paroxysmal pain
- Shooting pain through the area

Allodynia (painful hypersensitivity)
- Pain produced by light touch, particularly moving contact with skin
- Present in 90% of patients with postherpetic neuralgia
- Often very distressing
- Frequently, the last pain type to disappear, if at all

countries. However, the waning of immunity before adulthood has raised questions about the value of pediatric vaccination.

Adult VZV vaccination can be carried out in the 'at-risk' adult over 60 years to prevent VZV reactivation. A large randomized double-blind placebo-controlled trial (35 546 adults > 60 years) investigated vaccination with live attenuated VZV vaccine. The outcome was a reduction in the incidence of herpes zoster (59 vaccinations to prevent one case) and PHN (802 vaccinations to prevent one case). In immunocompromised recipients of bone marrow transplants, vaccination with an inactive VZV vaccine also reduces the incidence of PHN.

Antiviral treatment. If acute herpes zoster occurs, antiviral treatment should be given as soon as possible to reduce the severity and duration of the acute zoster episode and thus indirectly decrease the risk of PHN (there is no direct effect of antiviral treatment on PHN). Meta-analyses of RCTs have indicated that aciclovir (acyclovir) reduces the severity and duration of herpes zoster and acute zoster-associated pain. Aciclovir, 800 mg five times daily, should be given for 7 days. However, as the condition is often well established before treatment is started, antiviral therapy may be of limited effectiveness.

Effective pain treatment in the acute phase reduces risk of PHN. A 90-day course of amitriptyline, started during the acute herpes zoster attack, was found in an RCT to reduce pain intensity assessed 6 months later. Given the risk of side effects, TCAs should be used with caution in older patients; a trial of gabapentin or pregabalin may be preferable.

Pharmacological management of established PHN. Overall, pharmacological treatment of PHN tends to be unsatisfactory. It is not clear why some patients obtain good pain relief while others do not. It may reflect: different underlying mechanisms among patients despite similar initiating events; genetically determined variation in pain response (see Chapter 1); or differing influences of psychological and environmental factors.

Sympathetic blockade. Anecdotal observations of prompt pain reduction and apparent truncation of the evolution of acute shingles into PHN have led to the use of sympathetic blockade during the acute phase of this viral illness. However, supportive evidence from RCTs is lacking.

Systemic corticosteroids. Meta-analyses of RCTs show that corticosteroids do not prevent PHN.

Tricyclic antidepressants are useful for PHN, as in DN (see pages 95–6). SSRIs do not seem to be effective. SNRIs, although not studied in RCTs, are used clinically because of a smaller side-effect profile.

Anticonvulsants can effectively relieve postherpetic pain, as shown by meta-analyses of RCTs. The degree of effect is similar to that reported for DN (see pages 96–7). Gabapentin, pregabalin and sodium valproate have been reported to be effective in PHN. In a comparative study of gabapentin versus nortriptyline, pain relief results were similar, but gabapentin was better tolerated.

Capsaicin relieves pain associated with PHN. Capsaicin binds to vanilloid receptors on C and Aδ fibers, and provokes pain at initial application because of the release of substance P from the peripheral nerve terminals. This thermal cue makes blinding in RCTs difficult and may positively bias the benefits observed in such trials. Pain relief on repeated application of capsaicin reflects depletion of excitatory mediators from peripheral nerve endings.

Opioids. Discussion on the use of opioids in DN (see pages 97–8) applies equally to use in PHN or other neuropathic chronic pain.

Lidocaine skin patch. A meta-analysis of RCTs of topical lidocaine (lignocaine) patches for PHN reached no firm conclusion regarding effect.

Botulinum toxin. Injection of botulinum toxin for PHN has shown promise in one large clinical trial, although conclusive evidence from larger multicenter studies has yet to be reported.

Invasive approaches may need to be considered for severe neuropathic pain that does not respond to the usual treatments. Systemic lidocaine infusion may be used to bring a severe exacerbation of pain under control. Systemic ketamine infusion may be required in extreme situations.

In rare cases, a trial of spinal cord stimulation (SCS) may be warranted prior to considering permanent implantation of an SCS system – particularly in patients who are intolerant of drugs.

Non-pharmacological management. Trials to evaluate the effectiveness of transcutaneous electrical nerve stimulation (TENS) for chronic pain have been inconclusive owing to the small number of participants, a lack of placebo control, a lack of long-term assessment and inadequate details of the stimulation variables most likely to provide pain relief.

Since psychological stress generally activates and/or worsens neuropathic pain, no matter its etiology, treatment of psychological sequelae of PHN, such as anxiety and depression, as well as stress control in general, may improve a patient's ability to lead a normal life. Techniques such as 'cognitive-behavioral desensitization' (a strategy to reduce the emotional reactivity to neuropathic pain) may be invaluable.

Key points – diabetic and postherpetic neuropathic pain

- Persistent hyperglycemia is the primary factor responsible for nerve damage in diabetes mellitus. Diabetic neuropathy (DN) affects the autonomic and peripheral nervous systems.
- Maintenance of near-normal blood glucose levels is the best approach to primary and secondary prevention of DN.
- Tricyclic antidepressants (TCAs), serotonin–norepinephrine-reuptake inhibitors (SNRIs) and anticonvulsants are the medications of choice for neuropathic pain, but side effects are common. Pregabalin is specifically approved for DN. Duloxetine has also gained approval for DN in some countries.
- Combining medications that address different mechanisms (e.g. SNRIs or TCAs with gabapentinoids), while being mindful of drug interactions, can be helpful for treatment-resistant cases, and may enable smaller doses of one or both drugs to be given, which may reduce the total side-effect burden.
- Although efficacy in clinical trials is established, the use of opioids for the treatment of neuropathic pain remains controversial because of safety and overdose concerns, particularly in at-risk individuals, such as those with substance use disorder or psychiatric comorbidities, or those using benzodiazepines or other sedatives.
- Postherpetic neuralgia (PHN) is pain that persists after the vesicular rash of herpes zoster has resolved.
- During an attack of acute herpes zoster (shingles), reactivation of the varicella zoster virus (VZV), previously dormant in the dorsal root ganglia, induces inflammation and neuronal destruction.
- TCAs and anticonvulsants are useful therapies for PHN; the physical, psychological and social consequences of PHN should also receive attention.
- Once developed, PHN is difficult to manage and thus efforts to prevent PHN are crucial via: prevention of VZV infection, boosting VZV immunity, treating at the time of acute herpes zoster infection, and effective treatment of the acute pain.

Key references

Anon. Intensive blood-glucose control with sulphonylureas or insulin compared with conventional treatment and risk of complications in patients with type 2 diabetes (UKPDS 33). UK Prospective Diabetes Study (UKPDS) Group. *Lancet* 1998;352:837–53.

Boulton AJ, Vinik AI, Arezzo JC et al. Diabetic neuropathies: a statement by the American Diabetes Association. *Diabetes Care* 2005;28:956–62.

Cepeda MS, Farrar JT. Economic evaluation of oral treatments for neuropathic pain. *J Pain* 2006;7:119–28.

Chandra K, Shafiq N, Pandhi P et al. Gabapentin versus nortriptyline in post-herpetic neuralgia patients: a randomized, double-blind clinical trial—the GONIP trial. *Int J Clin Pharmacol Ther* 2006;44:358–63.

Collins SL, Moore RA, McQuay H, Wiffen P. Antidepressants and anticonvulsants for diabetic neuropathy and postherpetic neuralgia: a quantitative systematic review. *J Pain Symptom Manage* 2000;20:449–58.

Eisenberg E, McNicol ED, Carr DB. Efficacy and safety of opioid agonists in the treatment of neuropathic pain of nonmalignant origin: systematic review and meta-analysis of randomized controlled trials. *JAMA* 2005;293:3043–52.

Gajraj NM. Pregabalin: its pharmacology and use in pain management. *Anesth Analg* 2007;105:1805–15.

Gilron I, Bailey J et al. Nortriptylene and gabapentin, alone and in combination for neuropathic pain: a double-blind, randomized controlled crossover trial. *Lancet* 2009;374:1252–61.

Greene DA, Stevens MJ, Obrosova I, Feldman EL. Glucose-induced oxidative stress and programmed cell death in diabetic neuropathy. *Eur J Pharmacol* 1999;375:217–23.

Helgason S, Petursson G, Gudmundsson S, Sigurdsson JA. Prevalence of postherpetic neuralgia after a first episode of herpes zoster: prospective study with long term follow up. *BMJ* 2000;321:794–6.

Jung BF, Johnson RW, Griffin DR, Dworkin RH. Risk factors for postherpetic neuralgia in patients with herpes zoster. *Neurology* 2004;62:1545–51.

Kalso E, Edwards JE, Moore RA, McQuay HJ. Opioids in chronic non-cancer pain: systematic review of efficacy and safety. *Pain* 2004;112:372–80.

Kimberlin DW, Whitley RJ. Varicella-zoster vaccine for the prevention of herpes zoster. *N Engl J Med* 2007;356:1338–43.

Oxman MN, Levin MJ, Johnson GR et al. A vaccine to prevent herpes zoster and postherpetic neuralgia in older adults. *N Engl J Med* 2005;352:2271–84.

Santee JA. Corticosteroids for herpes zoster: what do they accomplish? *Am J Clin Dermatol* 2002;3:517–24.

Scobie IN, Samaras K. *Fast Facts: Diabetes Mellitus*, 3rd edn. Oxford: Health Press Limited, 2009.

Tolle T, Freynhagen R, Versavel M et al. Pregabalin for relief of neuropathic pain associated with diabetic neuropathy: a randomized, double-blind study. *Eur J Pain* 2008;12:203–13.

Wiffen P, Collins S, McQuay H et al. Anticonvulsant drugs for acute and chronic pain. *Cochrane Database Syst Rev* 2005;3:CD001133.

Woo EJ, Ball R, Braun MM. Varicella-zoster vaccine. *N Engl J Med* 2007;357:88.

Wood MJ, Kay R, Dworkin RH et al. Oral acyclovir therapy accelerates pain resolution in patients with herpes zoster: a meta-analysis of placebo-controlled trials. *Clin Infect Dis* 1996;22:341–7.

Xiao L, Mackey S, Hui H et al. Subcutaneous injection of botulinum toxin A is beneficial in postherpetic neuralgia. *Pain Med* 2010;11:1827–33.

7 Central pain

Central pain is defined by the International Association for the Study of Pain (IASP) as 'pain initiated or caused by a primary lesion (or dysfunction) of the central nervous system (CNS)'. It has been suggested that 'or dysfunction' be deleted, as peripheral nerve lesions can eventually lead to dysfunction in the CNS.

Spinal cord injury (SCI; trauma or disease) (Figure 7.1) and stroke are the most common causes of lesions in the spinal cord or brain and brainstem that cause central pain, but there are many others (Table 7.1). It has now been recognized that epilepsy can be painful as can Parkinson's disease. Multiple sclerosis causes central pain in about 60% of patients.

Pathophysiology

Post-stroke pain. Conditions sufficient for the generation of central pain were previously thought to be an imbalance between the spinothalamic

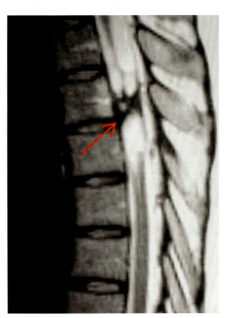

Figure 7.1 MRI scan showing spinal cord transection at the thoracic level secondary to trauma (see arrow). The patient suffered from paraplegia and spontaneous pain and allodynia in both legs.

TABLE 7.1
Sources of central pain

- Vascular lesions in the brain and spinal cord
- Infarction
- Hemorrhage
- Vascular malformation
- Multiple sclerosis
- Traumatic spinal cord injury
- Cordotomy
- Traumatic brain injury
- Syringomyelia and syringobulbia
- Tumors
- Abscesses
- Inflammatory diseases other than multiple sclerosis
- Myelitis caused by viruses or syphilis
- Epilepsy
- Parkinson's disease

From Wasner G, Baron R. Central pain syndromes. In: Castro-Lopes J, Raja S, Schmelz M, eds. *Pain 2008 – An Updated Review. IASP Refresher Course Syllabus.* Seattle: IASP Press, 2008.

system (caused by a lesion in that system) and medial lemniscal pathways. This is now known to be untrue. However, Craig et al. have provided evidence of a key role of ventromedial posterior thalamic lesions that allow disinhibition of a medial spinothalamic tract projecting via the medial dorsal nucleus of the thalamus to the anterior cingulate cortex (limbic system) – this appears to be associated with the burning nature of central post-stroke pain and also generates cold hypesthesia. In 2007, Kim et al. reported that lesions limited to the ventral caudal thalamic nucleus may produce a similar presentation of central post-stroke pain. Thus, there are several sites of lesion associated with post-stroke pain; unfortunately, this does not yet provide insight into the precise mechanisms of such pain.

Pain following spinal cord injury. The study of central pain arising from SCI has been more productive than that of post-stroke pain. Key insight was provided from a 5-year follow-up study of SCI pain by Siddall et al., which reported that at-level SCI pain often progressed to below-level pain – suggesting spinal and supraspinal mechanisms triggered by at-level SCI pain predispose to below-level 'central' pain.

A number of putative mechanisms have emerged from basic, clinical, epidemiological and brain-imaging research:
- loss of balance between different sensory channels
- loss of spinal inhibitory mechanisms
- presence of pattern generators above the level of SCI in the spinal cord or supraspinal relay nuclei
- synaptic plasticity changes
- spinal and supraspinal microglial activation (see Figure 1.8).

Brain-imaging studies have reported neuroplastic changes in the brain that correlate with the severity of post-SCI pain (see Figure 1.10).

Overall, complex processes appear to operate at the level of a 'spinal generator' and a 'supraspinal generator/amplifier'. The relative roles of each level in at-level and below-level SCI pain remain to be clarified. An important aspect is the relationship of post-SCI neuropathic pain and hyperreflexic responses (autonomic hyperreflexia). It has long been known that complete SCI lesions remove descending inhibitory control and allow severe autonomic mass reflexes. An example is severe vasoconstriction in response to a noxious stimulus – the vasoconstriction increases blood pressure which, in turn, activates vasomotor and other brainstem and brain structures, resulting in exacerbation of neuropathic pain (Figure 7.2).

Figure 7.2 Spinal cord injury, autonomic dysreflexia and pain. After a complete T4–6 transection, noxious stimulation below the lesion, such as a severely distended or infected bladder, results in a barrage of input to the spinal cord. (1) In the absence of any descending inhibitory processes an exaggerated sympathetic reflex response occurs, with vasoconstriction of gut vasculature; increased blood pressure activates baroreceptors and the brainstem vasomotor center, impinging on the periaqueductal gray (PAG) area that is a watershed for respiratory and hemodynamic control. Neuropathic pain perception increases as a result of these central changes. Also, vagal nerve activation results in compensatory bradycardia, nasal congestion, profuse sweating and flushing in the face and neck – as well as a pounding headache. (2) Noxious input to the cord also results in reflex activation of muscle without any normal inhibitory control (upper motor neuron lesion). Thus, spastic responses occur, which may be painful.

Diagnosis

Lesions in the brain. Stroke is the most common cause of neuropathic pain related to brain lesions. More than 8% of all patients who have had a stroke suffer with central pain. In view of the high incidence of stroke, about 90% of all central pain is associated with stroke. Because stroke is associated with communication difficulties, the high prevalence of central pain was not recognized until quite recently. Previously, it was erroneously believed that only thalamic lesions resulted in central pain. Now the diagnosis of 'thalamic syndrome' is

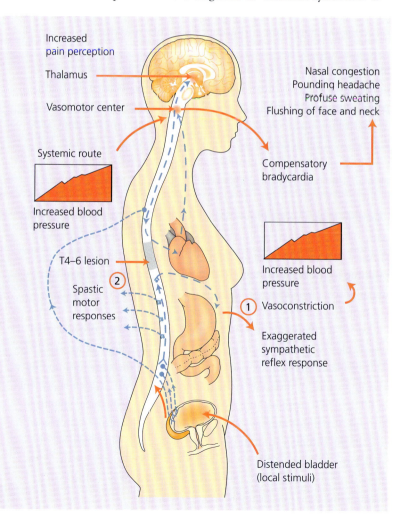

reserved for thalamic lesions and otherwise the diagnosis of 'post-stroke pain' is used.

Post-stroke pain is usually located within the area of loss of sensation caused by the stroke, though sometimes only part of the area is affected. Complex regional pain syndrome (CRPS) of the paretic arm may occur (see Chapter 5), but this is rare. Importantly, it has been suggested that some pain syndromes associated with stroke are initiated at the periphery; for example, nociceptive pain in the shoulder–arm due to subluxation of the scapulohumeral joint, neuropathic pain related to spasticity, and diabetic neuropathy reflecting the significant co-incidence of stroke and diabetes.

Spinal cord injury. Unfortunately, traumatic SCI is common, particularly in young men. In Europe, it is estimated that 300 000 people currently have SCI, with about 11 000 new cases per year. In a 5-year follow-up study in Australia, Siddall et al. reported that 34% had below-level neuropathic pain (see pain taxonomy, Table 7.2), which was deemed to be central pain. A further 41% had at-level neuropathic pain that probably started at the peripheral level, but usually became 'centralized'. Musculoskeletal and visceral pain contributed to an overall prevalence of 81% of participants reporting pain. There was a strong correlation between the presence of both types of neuropathic pain at 5 years and at earlier time points, pointing to the need to start treating the pain early to prevent the maladaptive changes described in Chapter 1, rather than 'waiting for the pain to go away'.

An IASP taxonomy of post-SCI pain types has been promulgated (see Table 7.2), based on an earlier proposal by Siddall et al. in 1997. This has facilitated comparison of studies using the same terminology. It is important to differentiate non-neuropathic pain, which is present in 60% of SCI patients at 5 years, and includes mechanical spinal instability, painful muscle spasms and secondary overuse syndromes (e.g. of the shoulder joint in paraplegics). Visceral pain may be associated with nociceptive visceral pathology, though in many cases no pathology is found and the pain is presumed to be below-level neuropathic pain (e.g. bladder and rectal pain).

TABLE 7.2
IASP taxonomy of pain following spinal cord injury

Broad type (tier one)	Broad system (tier two)	Specific structures and pathology (tier three)
Nociceptive	Musculoskeletal	Bone, joint, muscle trauma or inflammation
		Mechanical instability
		Muscle spasm
		Secondary or overuse syndrome
	Visceral	For example, renal calculus, bowel dysfunction, sphincter dysfunction
		Dysreflexic headache
Neuropathic	Above level	Compressive mononeuropathies
		Complex regional pain syndrome
	At level	Nerve root compression (including cauda equina)
		Syringomyelia
		Spinal cord trauma/ischemia (e.g. transitional zone)
		Dual-level cord and root trauma (double lesion syndrome)
	Below level	Spinal cord trauma/ischemia (e.g. central dysesthesia syndrome)

From Wasner G, Baron R. Central pain syndromes. In: Castro-Lopes J, Raja S, Schmelz M, eds. *Pain 2008 – An Updated Review. IASP Refresher Course Syllabus.* Seattle: IASP Press, 2008. IASP, International Association for the Study of Pain.

Onset of central pain

Time of pain onset after the initial lesion is extremely variable. In one study of SCI from trauma, 12% of patients had below-level neuropathic pain by 2 weeks after injury, and this had risen to 20%

by 6 months. However, the mean onset time (± implied standard deviation) was 1.8 ± 1.7 years (note the large variance). With stroke, 63% reported onset of central pain within 1 month, 19% between 1 and 6 months and another 19% between 6 and 12 months. Sometimes onset of central pain occurs several years after injury.

Pain sites
Central pain is usually localized in an area of complete or partial loss of sensation, or in an area of abnormal sensation. In SCI, pain may be on both sides of the body below the level of the spinal lesion. Sometimes all of the area below the level of the spinal lesion is painful, but in some patients the area may be smaller or even very localized (e.g. bladder or rectum).

Pain character
Usually, the neuropathic pain consists of sensations of continuous burning, aching and pricking. Spontaneous or evoked episodes of shooting or stabbing pain also often occur. Patients report that pain can be triggered by emotional situations and may be decreased by intense concentration on work or other mental activities. More than 70% of post-stroke patients suffer allodynia. Allodynia was found to be more common in incomplete SCI (compared with complete SCI) in the 2003 Siddall study.

There is no single pathognomonic description of central pain, though neuropathic descriptors can usually be elicited (see Chapter 2).

Treatment
Central pain is one of the most challenging of all chronic pain conditions. Except for a few exceptions, the underlying condition cannot be successfully treated. However, differential diagnosis of the type of pain is crucial to distinguish nociceptive pain and peripheral neuropathic pain from central pain (see Table 7.2).

The impact of central pain on the individual is usually severe, so a multidisciplinary assessment in a biopsychosocial framework is essential. In many cases a multimodal approach to treatment needs to incorporate pharmacological, psychological and physical therapy strategies. Invasive procedures may be needed in extreme cases.

Psychological, physical and other treatments. Physical therapy has a wide range of roles in patients with post-stroke and SCI pain because of complications related to immobility, postural changes and/or overuse syndromes, or to help relieve symptoms related to neurological disease, such as multiple sclerosis. Mirror visual feedback with 'virtual walking' was effective in 4 patients, but in another study imaginary ankle movement increased neuropathic pain in patients with SCI. Further research into such techniques is needed.

The use of cognitive behavioral therapy (CBT) has been evaluated in only one controlled study. At 12-month follow-up, patients receiving CBT had decreased levels of depression and anxiety but no change in pain. Control patients showed no changes.

Pharmacotherapy

Anticonvulsants. In 2008, Finnerup evaluated published randomized controlled trials in central pain with at least 10 participants. An anticonvulsant demonstrating efficacy in central pain in more than one study was pregabalin; those lacking evidence of efficacy were lamotrigine, sodium valproate and carbamazepine.

Antidepressants. A reduction in central post-stroke pain has been reported for amitriptyline, with the number needed to treat (NNT) being 1.7 (range 1–3) and pain-relieving effects noted from the second week of treatment onwards. The dosage of amitriptyline was increased from 12.5 mg twice daily up to 75 mg daily during the first week and then maintained at this level.

In contrast, there is no evidence for the efficacy of amitriptyline at doses of 50–125 mg in post-SCI central pain. However, there was evidence of an analgesic effect in a study of amitriptyline, 150 mg, in SCI pain, though the high dose raised concerns about potential cardiac toxicity. This suggests that trials of other less toxic medications with similar mechanisms, such as serotonin–norepinephrine-reuptake inhibitors (SNRIs) and, amongst the tricyclic antidepressants (TCAs), nortriptyline and desipramine, should be considered first.

Systemically administered local anesthetics. Some studies of intravenous lidocaine infusion report short-term efficacy for SCI pain or post-stroke pain. One study supports its use for SCI pain. A study of the oral analog of lidocaine, mexiletine, reported efficacy for SCI pain.

Intravenous anesthetics. A study of the γ-aminobutyric acid (GABA) agonist propofol, given intravenously, reported efficacy, though sedative effects complicated evaluation.

Intravenous ketamine has been reported to reduce continuous or evoked pain in small studies. However, Hocking and Cousins reported no evidence of long-term efficacy in any chronic pain condition when given by the oral route.

Cannabinoids. One study of the cannabinoid tetrahydrocannabinol (THC) at a dose of 10 mg reported efficacy in patients with multiple sclerosis. A second study reported an oromucosal spray based on whole-plant cannabis to be effective in relieving central pain.

Opioids. There is some evidence of short-term efficacy of opioids, but the long-term data that are available are not encouraging, with few patients persisting with opioid therapy.

Invasive procedures

Spinal cord stimulation has proven to be unsuccessful in the large majority of individuals with central pain. The only possible application lies in patients with Brown–Séquard syndrome (unilateral SCI) and pain in a limb with at least partially preserved sensation, which is rare.

Deep brain stimulation has not shown long-term efficacy. Motor cortex stimulation offers more encouraging results, but is still experimental.

Dorsal root entry zone (DREZ) lesioning involves a laminectomy to allow multiple radiofrequency lesions to be made in spinal cord dorsal horn substantia gelatinosa. This technique can provide complete pain relief for many years in patients with avulsion of the roots of the brachial plexus from the spinal cord. Strictly speaking this is a 'peripheral lesion'; however, often there is extensive damage to the spinal cord and the pain is similar to central pain. Patients of this type in whom pharmacotherapy fails should be considered for DREZ lesioning. To reduce the risk of serious complications, including paraplegia and/or extension of the

Key points – central pain

- Central pain results from lesions in the brain and brainstem or spinal cord. The most common causes are stroke and traumatic spinal cord injury (SCI), though there are many other causes.
- More than 8% of patients who have had a stroke develop central pain. This is probably an underestimate because communication problems may impede diagnosis of pain.
- Onset of post-stroke pain may occur up to several years after the injury.
- Within 2 weeks of SCI, 12% of patients have below-level neuropathic pain which is 'central'; by 6 months, 20% have central pain. Mean onset time is 1.8 ± 1.7 years (wide variation).
- The pathophysiology of central post-stroke pain (CPSP) involves a key role for lesions in diverse areas of the brain, including several different thalamic nuclei. One such lesion results in disinhibition of a nociceptive pathway that projects to the anterior cingulate cortex (limbic system) – this pathophysiology is associated with the burning quality of CPSP.
- The pathophysiology of SCI pain involves a 'spinal generator' and a 'supraspinal generator/amplifier'.
- Treatment of central pain is extremely challenging and requires a multimodal approach based on a biopsychosocial model. Differential diagnosis of pain type is crucial. New innovative physical/psychological treatments show promise of addressing maladaptive brain neuroplasticity changes.
- Pharmacotherapy, based on only a small number of controlled studies, have demonstrated efficacy of amitriptyline for CPSP (although not yet studied, a trial of serotonin–norepinephrine-reuptake inhibitors [SNRIs] may be preferable because of their lower toxicity) and pregabalin in both SCI and CPSP. Short-term efficacy has been reported for systemic (intravenous infusion) lidocaine (lignocaine), propofol and ketamine, but there is no evidence of long-term efficacy.
- Dorsal root entry zone lesioning can provide long-term relief of central pain after brachial plexus avulsion.

neurological deficit into the neck region, DREZ lesioning should be performed by a neurosurgeon with special training and experience.

Intrathecal drug administration. In SCI pain, one controlled study reported efficacy of morphine plus clonidine given intrathecally, but not for either drug alone. Even with the combination, only 50% of patients responded. Intrathecal baclofen relieves the muscle spasm and associated spasticity in SCI patients and may relieve pain associated with spasticity.

Key references

Andersen G, Vestergaard K, Ingeman-Nielsen M, Jensen TS. Incidence of central post-stroke pain. *Pain* 1995;61:187–93.

Craig AD, Bushnell MC, Zhang ET, Blomqvist A. A thalamic nucleus specific for pain and temperature sensation. *Nature* 1994;372:770–3.

Finnerup NB. Treatment of central pain. In: Castro-Lopec J, Rajas S, Schmelz M, eds. *Pain 2008. An Updated Review. Refresher Course Syllabus.* IASP Press, 2008:319–26.

Gustin SM, Wrigley PJ, Gandevia SC et al. Movement imagery increases pain in people with neuropathic pain following complete thoracic spinal cord injury. *Pain* 2008;137:237–44.

Henry JL, Panju A, Yashpal K, eds. *Central Neuropathic Pain: Focus on Post-Stroke Pain.* IASP Press, 2007.

Hocking G, Cousins MJ. Ketamine in chronic pain management: an evidence-based review. *Anesth Analg* 2003;97:1730–9.

Kim JH, Greenspan JD et al. Lesions limited to the human thalamic principal somatosensory nucleus (ventral caudal) are associated with loss of cold sensations and central pain. *J Neurosci* 2007;27:4995–5004.

Siddall PJ, Cousins MJ, Otte A et al. Pregabalin in central neuropathic pain associated with spinal cord injury: a placebo-controlled trial. *Neurology* 2006;67:1792–800.

Siddall PJ, McClelland JM, Rutkowski SB, Cousins MJ. A longitudinal study of the prevalence and characteristics of pain in the first 5 years following spinal cord injury. *Pain* 2003;103:249–57.

Siddall PJ, Molloy AR, Walker S et al. The efficacy of intrathecal morphine and clonidine in the treatment of pain after spinal cord injury. *Anesth Analg* 2000;91:1493–8.

Siddall PJ, Yezierski RP, Loeser JD. Taxonomy and epidemiology of spinal cord injury pain. In: Yezierski RP, Burchiel K, eds. *Spinal Cord Injury Pain: Assessment, Mechanisms, Management. Progress in Pain Research and Management Vol 23.* Seattle: IASP Press, 2002:9–24.

Yezierski RP. Spinal cord injury: a model for the pathophysiology and mechanisms of central pain. In: Castro-Lopec J, Rajas S, Schmelz M, eds. *Pain 2008. An Updated Review. Refresher Course Syllabus.* Seattle: IASP Press, 2008:307–17.

8 Persistent postsurgical pain

Persistent postsurgical pain

It is now clear from numerous studies that persistent postsurgical pain (PPSP) is one of the major causes of persistent (chronic) pain. Limited data also indicate that a significant percentage of patients continue to have pain following trauma, particularly trauma to multiple body areas or traumatic amputation.

Pathophysiology

Although there is evidence that nerve damage plays a key role, there are other factors that probably determine which patients with nerve damage progress from acute to persistent pain as, in many operations (e.g. amputation), all patients have nerve damage but only a percentage (10–50%) progress to chronic pain (Table 8.1). The only reliable data currently available derive from postsurgery patients and thus this discussion will be limited to these patients. It is possible, but not studied, that similar factors may occur in post-trauma patients

TABLE 8.1
Estimated incidence of persistent postsurgical pain following selected procedures

Procedure	Incidence of PPSP (%)
Amputation	30–50
Thoracotomy	20–50
Mastectomy	10–30
Major joint replacement	12
Hysterectomy	5–32
Inguinal hernia repair	5–10
Cesarean section	5–10

PPSP, persistent postsurgical pain.

(many of whom also undergo surgery). A major review of this subject by Kehlet et al. was published in 2006.

The factors in Table 8.2 are associated with increased risk of PPSP, but no comprehensive study has been carried out to evaluate their relative importance. Although evidence of genetic factors is not

TABLE 8.2
Factors contributing to the development of persistent postsurgical pain

Pre-existing pain
- Central nervous system hyperexcitability
- Opioid tolerance

Physical nerve injury
- Location of surgical procedure (for example, chest wall)
- Surgical technique

Postoperative pain severity
- Inadequate analgesia techniques
- Extent of tissue injury
- Psychological factors (for example, depression)
- Sex
- Genetics including pharmacogenetics

Impaired nerve repair (or aggravated injury)
- Radiotherapy
- Chemotherapy

Other factors
- Genetic
- Psychological (e.g. catastrophizing, depression)

From Macintyre P, Scott DA. Acute pain management and acute pain services. In: Cousins et al., 2009 (see Useful resources).

available for PPSP, Tegeder et al. (2006) have identified a genetic influence on the development of chronic pain following an acute episode of sciatica. More attention is now being focused on the influence of other patient factors, such as catastrophizing and depression, which influence perioperative and postoperative pain and analgesic use.

Prevention

Preoperative pain intensity has been correlated with postoperative pain intensity in a prospective study of 346 patients undergoing abdominal surgery. The intensity of postoperative pain has been linked to the prevalence of chronic pain. Thus, improved acute pain control pre- and postoperatively may help to prevent PPSP. There is also evidence that intra- and postoperative use of epidural or regional neural blockade may be helpful.

Surgical technique may play a role, as 'nerve preservation' techniques appear to lower the incidence of PPSP – although no studies have prospectively addressed this area. The introduction of video-assisted thoracic surgery made no difference to the incidence of post-thoracotomy PPSP at 1 year after surgery. This serves to illustrate how difficult it is to avoid trauma to nerves at various surgical sites, and that factors other than nerve injury are involved in PPSP.

Treatment

In the early stages of PPSP surgeons tend to suspect a surgical complication of some sort (e.g. a wound hematoma, chronic infection, incomplete repair of an inguinal hernia). Initially, a reasonable attempt should be made to rule out such diagnoses. However, in the majority of cases no remediable surgical complication will be found. Recognition that the patient has chronic pain, and that the pathophysiology is in the central nervous system, not in the peripheral tissues, is now needed.

Patient education. As the majority of PPSP is caused by nerve damage, the treatment options are similar to those for other neuropathic pain syndromes. Pharmacotherapy alone will rarely be sufficient. A biopsychosocial assessment should be made and treatment plans should aim to rectify maladaptive changes in physical, psychological and environmental domains. For example, patients are rarely told that PPSP is a possible complication of surgery. Thus, patients often feel angry and let down and find it difficult to move on unless the anger is addressed with careful explanation and reassurance. Patients may have been stigmatized at work because of a perceived unnecessarily long recovery, requiring input to the workplace. Preoperative patient education about the possibility of PPSP, during the informed consent procedure, may reduce the negative postoperative psychosocial consequences that can complicate treatment. In the authors' experience of patients with PPSP, and supported by several studies, psychosocial factors such as catastrophizing and the pain itself often activate stress and mood disorders, thus worsening pain and interfering with adaptive coping.

Pharmacotherapy relies on tricyclic antidepressants (TCAs), serotonin–norepinephrine-reuptake inhibitors (SNRIs), anticonvulsants and sometimes membrane stabilizers. In severe cases a trial of subcutaneous peripheral nerve stimulation (PNS) may be necessary. PNS is emerging as a valuable option for postinguinal hernia repair PPSP. In a trial stimulation, electrodes are placed across the path of ilio-inguinal, iliohypogastric and genitofemoral nerves; if the trial stimulation is successful patients proceed at a later date to implantation of electrodes and a pulse generator.

Postincisional pain

Postincisional syndrome is defined as pain at or close to the site of a surgical incision that persists beyond the usual healing period. As with other neuropathic pain syndromes, patients exhibit allodynia and sometimes also edema in the vicinity of the surgical wound, which is typical of temporary peripheral sensitization.

Postamputation persistent pain

Postamputation persistent pain is a special case of PPSP because large nerves are deliberately cut in all patients. It is interesting, then, that only 30–50% develop PPSP, whereas 100% have nerve injury (see Table 8.1).

This emphasizes the multifactorial basis of PPSP. A surprising omission in studies of amputation pain is information about how the nerves amputated are managed (i.e. clean cut or ligature tied). Use of a ligature tie in animal studies is known to generate neuropathic pain.

The clinical context of amputation may play a role. For example, when the amputation occurs because of a progressive disease, such as diabetes, disease-related preoperative nerve damage and pain are involved. Conversely, traumatic amputation or amputation to prevent spread of disease, such as in breast cancer, may not involve prior nerve damage or pain.

Pathophysiology. The neuromas that form at the end of cut nerves after amputation are hypersensitive and have abnormally dense sodium (and other ion) channels that generate ectopic discharges. This abnormal activity initiates and maintains the central sensitization associated with nerve injury (see Chapter 1). There may also be a change in the distribution of sodium channel subtypes, with an upregulation of $Na_V1.8$. This opens up a possible new selective target, as $Na_V1.8$ occurs only on small primary afferent fibers. As with central pain, after amputation there is synaptic reorganization in the spinal cord, brainstem, thalamus and primary somatosensory cortex, which becomes newly responsive to neighboring body parts. These changes contribute to the persistent pain experienced after amputation.

Diagnosis. Phantom experiences, phantom pain and stump pain are different entities that share the same pathophysiological mechanisms. A phantom experience is a non-painful sensation; phantom pain is pain in an absent body part; and stump pain is local pain in the residual limb (i.e. at the amputation site). Up to 96% of amputees report phantom experiences, and 49% complain of stump pain. Depending on the tissue amputated, phantom pain may have an early prevalence in excess of 50%. Phantom pain affects not only limbs; phantom bladder, rectal, penile, breast and vaginal pain after surgery are all well described.

While phantom sensations may be described as tingling or itchy, phantom pain consists primarily of burning, cramping and shooting pains. Phantom sensations and phantom pain typically begin within days of the amputation, and tend to decrease in frequency and duration over time, though they persist for years in 40% of amputees. Sometimes phantom pain in the missing body part is similar to the pain present before the amputation.

Prevention. To date, attempts to prevent the development of phantom pain using peridural anesthesia or regional blocks have not proven successful. However, the randomized controlled trials (RCTs) that have evaluated these preventive regimens have not uniformly suppressed afferent input from the involved site. Therefore, the results of the studies should be interpreted as inconclusive rather than negative.

Treatment
Ketamine, a non-competitive N-methyl D-aspartate (NMDA) receptor antagonist, has been used in humans to treat various neuropathic pain syndromes. Intravenous ketamine provides relief from phantom and stump pain, but one small crossover RCT indicated a high incidence of side effects.

Opioids. Small randomized studies have suggested that morphine decreases pain intensity, albeit during short-term observation periods.

Antidepressants and anticonvulsants. There is a scarcity of controlled trial results to guide clinicians in the treatment of phantom pain, and clinicians must rely on favorable results from clinical research in which these agents have been given to treat other neuropathic pain syndromes.

Mirror therapy, which is based on manipulating neuroplastic changes in the brain associated with phantom pain, has been reported to reduce phantom limb pain in clinical reports and in a small RCT in which it was significantly more effective ($p = 0.008$) for reducing pain than guided imagery and sham mirror therapy.

Neurostimulation of various types (low- and high-intensity transcutaneous electrical nerve stimulation [TENS], transcranial magnetic stimulation of the motor cortex, epidural cervical spinal cord stimulation and epidural motor cortex stimulation) has been reported to be effective for phantom pain in case series, though carefully controlled trials have yet to be performed.

Key points – persistent postsurgical pain

- Persistent postsurgical pain (PPSP) is defined as pain at or close to the site of surgical incision that persists beyond the expected healing period.
- The incidence of PPSP varies from about 10% for very limited peripheral surgery, such as inguinal hernia repair or joint replacement, to 10–30% for mastectomy and up to 50% for thoracotomy and amputation.
- Nerve injury plays an important role in pathogenesis, but genetics, pre-existing pain and severity of postoperative pain are also risk factors, in addition to cancer treatment and possible psychosocial factors.
- Patients who catastrophize, which increases postoperative pain and opioid analgesic use, may benefit from psychological services such as cognitive behavioral therapy.
- Effective acute pain control may be preventive for PPSP – for example, intra- and postoperative use of epidural analgesia can prevent PPSP following some operations.
- Pharmacotherapy is based on the study results of neuropathic drugs used to treat pain caused by other types of nerve injury. Tricyclic antidepressants and anticonvulsants are first-line drugs.
- Peripheral nerve stimulation is emerging as a possible treatment option for severe PPSP.
- Although spinal cord stimulation (SCS) has not been found to be successful for amputation pain, early data indicate positive outcomes for dorsal root (DRG) stimulation.

Key references

Aasvang EK, Brandsborg B, Christensen B et al. Neurophysiological characterization of postherniotomy pain. *Pain* 2008;137:173–81.

Aasvang E, Kehlet H. Chronic postoperative pain: the case of inguinal herniorrhaphy. *Br J Anaesth* 2005;95:69–76.

Brandsborg B, Nikolajsen L, Hansen CT et al. Risk factors for chronic pain after hysterectomy: a nationwide questionnaire and database study. *Anesthesiology* 2007;106:1003–12.

Brennan TJ, Kehlet H. Preventive analgesia to reduce wound hyperalgesia and persistent postsurgical pain: not an easy path. *Anesthesiology* 2005;103:681–3.

Bruce J, Drury N, Poobalan AS et al. The prevalence of chronic chest and leg pain following cardiac surgery: a historical cohort study. *Pain* 2003;104:265–73.

Chan BL, Witt R, Charrow AP et al. Mirror therapy for phantom limb pain. *N Engl J Med* 2007;357:2206–7.

Cruccu G, Aziz TZ, Garcia-Larrea L et al. EFNS guidelines on neurostimulation therapy for neuropathic pain. *Eur J Neurol* 2007;14:952–70.

Jouguelet-Lacoste J, La Colla L, Schilling D, Chelly JE. The use of intravenous infusion or single dose of low-dose ketamine for postoperative analgesia: a review of the current literature. *Pain Med* 2015;16:383–403.

Jung BF, Ahrendt GM, Oaklander AL, Dworkin RH. Neuropathic pain following breast cancer surgery: proposed classification and research update. *Pain* 2003;104:1–13.

Kahn RS, Ahmed K, Blakeway E et al. Catastrophizing: a predictive factor for postoperative pain. *Am J Surg* 2011;201:122–31.

Kehlet H. Chronic pain after groin hernia repair. *Br J Surg* 2008;95:135–6.

Kehlet H, Jensen TS, Woolf CJ. Persistent postsurgical pain: risk factors and prevention. *Lancet* 2006;367:1618–25.

Kent ML, Tighe PJ, Belfer I et al. The ACTTION-APS-AAPM pain taxonomy (AAAPT) multidimensional approach to classifying acute pain conditions. *Pain Med* 2017;18:947–58.

McCormick Z, Chang-Chien G, Marshall B et al. Phantom limb pain: a systematic neuroanatomical-based review of pharmacologic treatment. *Pain Med* 2014;15:292–305.

Nikolajsen L, Brandsborg B, Lucht U et al. Chronic pain following total hip arthroplasty: a nationwide questionnaire study. *Acta Anaesthesiol Scand* 2006;50:495–500.

Nikolajsen L, Sorensen HC, Jensen TS, Kehlet H. Chronic pain following Caesarean section. *Acta Anaesthesiol Scand* 2004;48:111–16.

Riddle DL, Wade JB, Jiranek WA, Kong X. Preoperative pain catastrophizing predicts pain outcome after knee arthroplasty. *Clin Orthop Relat Res* 2010;468:798–806.

Tegeder I, Costigan M, Griffin RS et al. GTP cyclohydrolase and tetrahydrobiopterin regulate pain sensitivity and persistence. *Nat Med* 2006;12:1269–77.

Theunissen M, Peters ML, Bruce J et al. Preoperative anxiety and catastrophizing: a systematic review and meta-analysis of the association with chronic postsurgical pain. *Clin J Pain* 2012;28:819–41.

Upp J, Kent M, Tighe PJ. The evolution and practice of acute pain medicine. *Pain Med* 2013;14:124–44.

Young Casey C, Greenberg MA, Nicassio PM et al. Transition from acute to chronic pain and disability: a model including cognitive, affective, and trauma factors. *Pain* 2008;134:69–79.

9 Cancer pain

Pain in patients with cancer may present as various types of pain at different stages of the patient's journey with cancer. Thus, the pain may comprise acute, recurrent or chronic presentations due to the cancer and/or its treatment. Assessment of pain in patients with cancer should be the same as in other patients with pain (see Chapter 2), so that the widest possible range of treatments can be considered, with the aim of optimal treatment. Other additional symptoms such as fatigue, nausea, anxiety, depression, breathlessness and insomnia are common and also require treatment. Also, patients with cancer may have pre-existing chronic pain that continues, in addition to cancer pain (Table 9.1). Some patients with aggressive tumors may have escalating (or 'crescendo') pain requiring optimum pain management options, and

TABLE 9.1
Types of pain in patients with cancer

- Patients with acute cancer-related pain
  - associated with the diagnosis of cancer
  - associated with cancer therapy (surgery, chemotherapy or radiation)
- Patients with chronic cancer-related pain
  - associated with cancer progression
  - associated with cancer therapy (surgery, chemotherapy or radiation)
- Patients with pre-existing chronic pain and cancer-related pain
- Patients with a history of drug addiction and cancer-related pain
  - actively involved in illicit drug use
  - in methadone maintenance programs
  - with a history of drug abuse
- Dying patients with cancer-related pain

the needs of cancer 'survivors' – who live for many years with chronic pain and who are increasing in numbers – also need to be addressed. Finally, patients with cancer require particular strategies during the end-of-life stage. The choice of treatment options is based on similar considerations to those for patients with chronic non-cancer pain.

Unfortunately, the prevalence of pain is high in patients with cancer: 20–50% at the time of diagnosis; 50% during the treatment phase; 75–90% during the advanced cancer phase. At all of these stages, still less than 50% of patients receive effective pain relief according to studies in the USA, France and China – despite the fact that use of the *full range* of currently available options could provide relief for over 90% of patients. Sadly, this lamentable situation is no better for children: a study in Australia in 2010 reported that treatment was successful in only 47% of children.

Many studies report that unrelieved cancer pain is associated with interference with several dimensions of quality of life of the patients and their caregivers. Prevalence and severity of pain may be lower in hematologic malignancies such as lymphomas and leukemias compared with solid tumors such as breast and prostate cancers, which commonly metastasize to bone as well as invading nerve plexuses. However, variability in presentation of pain and its treatment (see Tables 9.1 and 9.2) make it essential to carefully evaluate each patient regardless of the cancer type.

Pathophysiology

Acute pain occurs in patients with cancer after surgery, radiotherapy or chemotherapy. After one or more of these treatments is finished, a percentage of patients progress to persistent pain (chronic pain), often caused by nerve damage from the treatments themselves. Risk factors in patients after cancer surgery are similar to those for any surgery (see Table 8.2). The incidence of such pain is given in Table 8.1. It is likely that the risk of persistent pain is higher in patients who also receive radiotherapy and/or chemotherapy, in addition to surgery.

The large majority of episodes of acute cancer-related pain are due to tumor invasion of pain-sensitive structures, which causes pathophysiological processes of the 'injury response', including inflammation, edema, acidosis and necrosis. Specific pathophysiological mechanisms are listed in Table 9.2.

Many such pains improve with treatment of the cancer, but some will proceed to a chronic version of the acute presentation (Tables 9.2–9.5).

Chronic pain may be caused directly by the cancer (about 78%), treatment of the cancer (19%), or conditions unrelated to the cancer (e.g. concurrent diseases) and/or factors in the psychosocial domains (3%) (see Tables 9.2–9.5). However, many patients have multiple pain

TABLE 9.2

Pain syndromes in patients with cancer: pain directly caused by cancer (primary or metastatic)

Mechanism	Characteristics of pain
Infiltration of bone by tumor ± fracture	Dull constant ache ± muscle spasm, with increased pain on movement
Infiltration or compression of nerve tissue by tumor	Burning constant pain in area of sensory loss ± hyperalgesia ± paroxysmal pain
Obstruction of hollow viscus	Poorly localized dull deep sickening pain with superficial hyperalgesia over referred surface area
Occlusion of arteries and veins by tumor	Ischemic pain in skin or claudication (muscle) ± signs of ischemia or venous engorgement
Stretching of periosteum or fascia – in tissues with tight investment	Severe localized pain (periosteum) or typical visceral pain (e.g. ovary)
Inflammation, owing to necrosis and infection	Severe localized pain and signs of tumor infection (± superficial ulceration)
Soft tissue infiltration	Localized pain, foul-smelling if ulcerated
Raised intracranial pressure	Severe constant headache, confusion etc.
Spinal cord compression	Severe back pain – worse at night
	Subtle sensory changes initially, motor and sensory deficits eventually
	Urinary bladder control impaired

TABLE 9.3
Pain associated with cancer therapy

Mechanism	Examples
Following surgery	Acute postoperative pain
	Neuropathic pain due to nerve damage or amputation
Following radiotherapy	Acute nerve lesions
	Chronic radiation fibrosis causing nerve damage
	Myelopathy of spinal cord
	Peripheral nerve lesions
Following chemotherapy	Peripheral neuropathy in hands and feet
	Steroid-induced pseudorheumatism in multiple joints
	Aseptic necrosis due to steroids (in femoral or humoral head)
	Postherpetic neuralgia

TABLE 9.4
Pain from comorbid conditions

Mechanism	Common sites and pain characteristics
Neuropathy (e.g. diabetic)	Burning pain in hands, feet
Degenerative disk disease	Back pain ± radicular pain
Rheumatoid arthritis	Joint pain on movement
Diffuse osteoporosis	Back pain, limb pain
Posture abnormalities	Back pain, muscle spasm etc. with depression, after surgery etc.
Myofascial pain syndromes	Local muscle pain ± spasm
Headache	Tension type or migraine

TABLE 9.5

Psychological comorbidities augmenting pain

Psychological factor	Possible causes
Anxiety	Sleeplessness
	Fear of death; loss of dignity (loss of self-control)
	Fear of surgical mutilation; uncontrollable pain
	Fear of the future; loss of social position and work
	Confused understanding of disease owing to poor communication
	Family and financial problems
Depression	Sleeplessness
	Loss of physical abilities
	Sense of helplessness
	Disfigurement
	Loss of valued social position, financial problems
Anger	Frustration with therapeutic failures
	Resentment of sickness
	Irritability caused by pain and general discomfort

A vicious 'circle' usually develops:

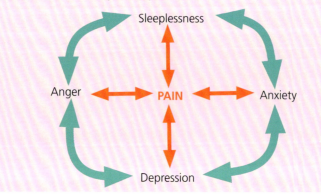

sites and pain types: for example, a high percentage (30–40%) have muscle pain in addition to cancer-related pain.

Diagnosing non-cancer pain is important as it emphasizes to patients the lack of a one-to-one relationship between the stage of cancer and the presence and severity of pain. However, Gonzales et al. (1991) found that, in 18% of patients presenting with pain as a problem, a thorough history and examination revealed new evidence of metastatic disease requiring anti-tumor treatment.

Metastatic spread of cancer to bone is the most common cause of cancer pain (Figure 9.1). Animal models using mice that had sarcoma cells implanted into the femur showed pain behavior related both to bone destruction and to the release of inflammatory mediators derived from the tumor (e.g. prostaglandins, cytokines, endothelins). Macrophages, which are often present in large numbers in some tumor masses, also produce mediators such as tumor necrosis factor and interleukins capable of activating nociceptors (see Chapter 1).

Yet chronic cancer pain is a nociceptive mosaic; pain may be due to tumor infiltration of nerves (neuropathic pain) or other tissues

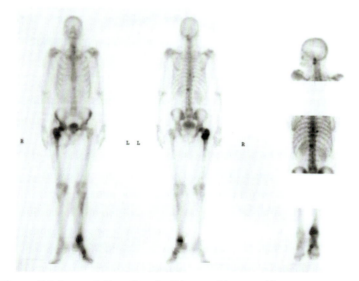

Figure 9.1 Bone scintigraphy of a 54-year-old man with prostate cancer and bone metastases. The scans show increased uptake at the sites of metastases in the cervical and lumbar spine, femur, tibia and metatarsal bone.

(somatic or visceral pain), or may be related to the treatment or procedure that the patient receives. Given the spectrum of potential pain sources and mechanisms, it is clear that several elements may be active in a single patient with cancer pain and that treatment should address all the pain mechanisms at play (Tables 9.2–9.5). Thus, regardless of the initial cause of pain, central sensitization can play a key role in cancer pain (see Chapter 1). Also neuroplastic changes may occur in the brain (see Chapter 1).

As with all chronic pain, psychosocial factors are of profound importance in patients with cancer pain (see Table 9.5). Saunders' concept of 'total pain' encompasses all of the factors that may affect the pain experienced by patients with cancer, including physical, psychological, social and spiritual elements.

Assessment

The same principles of pain assessment as described in Chapter 2 apply to patients with cancer pain. However, in this scenario, it is crucial to establish whether the pain is related to the cancer itself, the associated treatments or other conditions (see Tables 9.2–9.5).

Thus, patients should be asked about the onset of pain – whether it was present before the cancer or associated with the initiation of treatments such as surgery, chemotherapy or radiotherapy – and whether it has progressed. An oncological history must be added to the general medical component of the patient's history. The findings of a new physical examination may suggest a relapse or the interim development of new metastases that would warrant further investigation, so CT scans, MRI and other investigations are more readily ordered for cancer patients than for non-cancer patients.

Efforts should be made to identify the specific underlying pain syndrome, as the different types may respond differently to various analgesic therapies (Tables 9.1–9.5). In addition, open discussions with patients and their families about concerns and misconceptions surrounding the use of opioids should take place early on, as opioids are the treatment of choice for moderate to severe cancer pain.

Table 9.6 summarizes the aspects of assessment that require particular emphasis in patients with cancer.

TABLE 9.6
Essential aspects of assessment in patients with cancer

- Disease status and current treatments – implications for pain treatment options
- Pain 'experience' (e.g. PQRSTU; see Table 2.1)
- Current and previous management of pain and other symptoms
- Other associated symptoms, e.g. nausea, vomiting, dyspnea, fatigue
- Pain *meaning* for the patient and beliefs/knowledge
- Cognitive assessment
- Psychosocial assessment
- Physical examination – often multiple systems examined, particularly if metastases are present; further investigations may be needed
- Functional status evaluation
- Risk factors for poorly controlled pain or opioid abuse
- Patient preferences in view of goals (particular priorities) and expectations of pain treatment; advance directives etc.
- Be alert to oncological emergencies (e.g. acute spinal cord compression)

Treatment

A personalized mechanism-based stepped care model has emerged as the foundational concept of effective cancer pain management, much like for all chronic pain care (see Chapter 3). Opioids are now considered just one, albeit crucial, therapeutic tool in a multimodal approach that includes mechanism-based pharmacology, psychosocial, integrative, physical, pharmacological, neuromodulatory and neural blockade interventional procedures, combined according to each individual patient's evolving clinical course and need. A comprehensive assessment (see Chapter 2 and Table 9.6) is essential in identifying the basis of the pain in individual cancer patients (Tables 9.2–9.5). The key to effective management lies in choosing from one or more treatments, rather than relying only on one option such as pharmacological management. This is particularly important for 'cancer survivors' with chronic pain.

Many of the preceding chapters describe pain conditions and treatments that are applicable to both non-cancer pain and cancer pain, with treatments in the areas of pharmacology, physical therapy, psychological strategies, interventional treatments and other options.

The main treatments for cancer pain are summarized in Chapter 3:
- patient education about pain
- self-help 'active' strategies
- cognitive behavioral treatment (CBT)
- relaxation/meditation
- pharmacotherapy
- invasive procedures (interventional approaches).

Treatment of the cancer itself. In addition, if feasible, treatment of the cancer itself, with chemotherapy, surgery, external radiotherapy and/or radionuclide therapy is potentially a primary option for reducing pain. Conversely, each of these treatment options can be the cause of further pain – usually neuropathic (see Table 9.3). Thus, there needs to be a detailed discussion about the risks and benefits of treatment.

External radiotherapy employs ionizing radiation to destroy cancer cells. A systematic review of randomized controlled trials (RCTs) found that radiation is efficacious to treat pain from bone metastasis. The trial data indicate that 1 of every 4 individuals treated with external radiotherapy experiences 50% pain relief within 1 month.

Radiation therapy produces pain relief by inducing apoptotic death, not only of tumor cells, thereby reducing pressure in the bone marrow, but also of highly radiosensitive inflammatory cells. The multifraction regimen is the most widely used (i.e. 30 Gy delivered in ten treatment fractions over 2 weeks). However, no particular fractionation schedule has been found to be superior.

Radionuclide therapy is the systemic use of radioisotopes; it is a form of internal radiotherapy. Radioisotopes produce pain relief with a similar degree, onset and duration as radiotherapy. However, thrombocytopenia and neutropenia are common toxic effects of radioisotopes.

A systematic review of RCTs has found that a combination of strontium radioisotopes and radiotherapy produces better quality of life scores than radiotherapy alone.

Key points – cancer pain

- Cancer pain is a nociceptive mosaic in which pain may arise from inflammation, tumor infiltration of nerves (neuropathic pain) or other tissues (visceral or somatic pain), treatment, diagnostic and therapeutic procedures, and from other psychological and environmental factors.
- Treatment of the cancer itself (by chemotherapy, radiotherapy, surgery etc.) is a primary option in cancer pain management; however, such treatment may be the cause of pain (especially neuropathic pain).
- Opioids are the foundation for management of cancer pain of moderate to severe intensity, but other drugs should also be considered depending on the pain conditions and mechanisms involved (e.g. neuropathic, myofascial, arthritic); however, treatment of cancer pain should not rely on drugs alone, since there are many other options that will produce good results.
- Psychological therapies that promote 'self-help' strategies, such as cognitive behavioral therapy (CBT) and meditation/relaxation, as well as integrative treatments such as massage and acupuncture, are often useful as part of a multimodal treatment approach to support patients with cancer pain and related symptoms.
- Radiotherapy is effective for pain from bone metastases.
- Neural blockade can be used for isolated pain-causing lesions.

Key references

Bennett MI, Bagnall AM, Jose Closs S. How effective are patient-based educational interventions in the management of cancer pain? Systematic review and meta-analysis. *Pain* 2009;143:192–9.

Berenson J, Pflugmacher R, Jarzem P et al. Balloon kyphoplasty versus non-surgical fracture management for treatment of painful vertebral body compression fractures in patients with cancer: a multicentre, randomised controlled trial. *Lancet Oncol* 2011;12:225–35.

Boyd C, Crawford C, Paat CF et al. The impact of massage therapy on function in pain populations – a systematic review and meta-analysis of randomized controlled trials: part II, cancer pain populations. *Pain Med* 2016;17:1553–68.

Cousins MJ, Lynch ME. The declaration of Montreal: access to pain management is a fundamental human right. *Pain* 2011;152:2673–4.

Crespin DJ, Griffin KH, Johnson JR et al. Acupuncture provides short-term pain relief for patients in a total joint replacement program. *Pain Med* 2015;16:1195–203.

Gonzales GR, Elliott KJ, Portenoy RK, Foley KM. The impact of a comprehensive evaluation in the management of cancer pain. *Pain* 1991;47:141–4.

Mao JJ, Bowman MA, Xie SX et al. Electroacupuncture versus gabapentin for hot flashes among breast cancer survivors: a randomized placebo-controlled trial. *J Clin Oncol* 2015;33:3615–20.

McNicol E, Strassels SA, Goudas L et al. NSAIDs or paracetamol, alone or combined with opioids, for cancer pain. *Cochrane Database Syst Rev* 2005;2:CD005180.

Raphael J, Ahmedzai S, Hester J et al. Cancer pain: part 1: pathophysiology; oncological, pharmacological, and psychological treatments: a perspective from the British Pain Society. *Pain Med* 2010;11:742–64.

Raphael J, Hester J, Ahmedzai et al. Cancer pain: part 2: physical, interventional and complimentary therapies; management in the community; acute, treatment-related and complex cancer pain: a perspective from the British Pain Society. *Pain Med* 2010;11: 872–96.

Ripamonti CI, Santini D, Maranzano E et al. Management of cancer pain: ESMO Clinical Practice Guidelines. *Ann Oncol* 2012;23(Suppl 7):vii139–54.

Saunders CM. *Management of Terminal Malignant Disease*, 1st edn. London: Edward Arnold, 1978.

Smith TJ, Coyne PJ, Staats PS et al. An implantable drug delivery system (IDDS) for refractory cancer pain provides sustained pain control, less drug-related toxicity, and possibly better survival compared with comprehensive medical management (CMM). *Ann Oncol* 2005;16:825–33.

Swarm RA, Karanikolas M, Rao LK, Cousins MJ. Interventional approaches for chronic pain. In: *Oxford Textbook of Palliative Medicine*, 4th edn. Oxford: Oxford University Press, 2015:ch.9.8.

Wolfe J, Grier HE, Klar N et al. Symptoms and suffering at the end of life in children with cancer. *N Engl J Med* 2000;342:326–33.

Wong R, Wiffen PJ. Bisphosphonates for the relief of pain secondary to bone metastases. *Cochrane Database Syst Rev* 2002;2:CD002068.

Yates P, Edwards H, Nash R et al. A randomized controlled trial of a nurse-administered educational intervention for improving cancer pain management in ambulatory settings. *Patient Educ Couns* 2004;53:227–37.

10 Musculoskeletal pain

Chronic low back pain

Chronic back pain is defined by orthopedic surgeons as back pain that lasts longer than 7–12 weeks. Frequent recurring back pain is also classified as chronic pain, as it intermittently affects an individual over a long period. Chronic back pain has also been defined as pain that lasts beyond the expected period of healing. Furthermore, insurance and industrial sources consider individuals to have chronic back pain if their symptoms result in loss of work or disability. In recent studies examining burden of disease, the number one condition associated with the most years lived with disability was low back pain. Data from Australia and worldwide have demonstrated similar results (see Introduction).

Given this variety of definitions, estimates of prevalence vary (Table 10.1). In contrast to the prevalence of osteoarthritis (see page 154), that of back pain decreases with age (see Table 10.1). One epidemiological study in the Netherlands found that as many as 25% of individuals with new-onset low back pain were symptomatic at 12 months, though in most cases pain resolved within 2 months. Symptoms of pain in the lower back are more prevalent than those in the mid or upper back.

TABLE 10.1

Estimates of prevalence for chronic low back pain

Prevalence	Range (%)
Point	12–33
1 year	22–65
Lifetime	11–84
In people aged < 80 years	14–51
In people aged ≥ 80 years	7–22

Pathophysiology. Chronic low back pain is a complex biopsychosocial process that cannot be explained on purely anatomic, biomechanical, neurophysiological, immunologic, inflammatory or neurochemical grounds. For example, job dissatisfaction and fear of re-injury are strong risk factors for the development of chronic pain in individuals with acute back pain. Low income and poor education are also risk factors for chronic back pain and disability, possibly related to physical and psychological stressors of lower income jobs associated with low education. For these reasons some researchers argue that chronic disability from back pain is primarily related to a psychosocial dysfunction, but the validity and reliability of this statement is uncertain.

Models of low back pain indicate that mechanical and neurochemical factors interact closely. Mechanical trauma could lead to the production of metalloproteinases and cytokines; the actions of these substances on the extracellular matrix of the intervertebral disk produce disk degeneration and pain.

When the etiology of low back pain is apparent, there is most often a musculoskeletal abnormality of the lumbar spine, such as muscle strain, arthritis or disk degeneration or facet joint arthropathy. Back pain may also be accompanied by radiating pain in a radicular pattern into the lower limb due to nerve root irritation or compression (often called 'sciatica'). Low back pain may also be referred from visceral pathology, including vascular problems such as abdominal aortic aneurysm and cancer.

Like other chronic pain syndromes, chronic back pain may also involve central neuroplastic changes such as neuronal hyperactivity, changes in membrane excitability and expression of new genes that perpetuate pain even in the absence of new tissue injury.

Diagnosis of chronic back pain is a clinical one. Although anatomic abnormalities can be readily identified by imaging studies, there is no causal relationship between radiographic findings and non-specific low back pain, because most radiological abnormalities are common in asymptomatic people. Careful physical examination may help isolate anatomic contributions to low back pain, but often it is difficult to reach a specific diagnostic formulation.

The diagnostic strategy recommended by the US Agency for Healthcare Policy and Research in 1994 (now the Agency for Healthcare Research and Quality) remains valid today. It is appropriate to start symptomatic therapy without imaging in adults under 50 years of age who lack so-called 'red flags' – signs or symptoms of systemic disease or progressive neurological dysfunction indicating tumor, abscess, fracture or cauda equina syndrome.

For patients over 50 years of age, or for those whose history or physical findings raise the possibility of 'red flags', plain radiography and simple laboratory tests can almost completely rule out any serious underlying conditions such as fracture, cancer or abscess.

Indications for MRI or CT are shown in Table 10.2. Although physicians and patients prefer MRI to radiographic evaluations, MRI offers little additional benefit to patients. In fact, the use of MRI may elevate the costs of care because of the increased number of unnecessary spine operations.

If pain is not substantially improved within 6 weeks, further diagnostic evaluation is appropriate; the choice of imaging study depends on the clinical syndrome. Although MRI is a logical next step, CT scanning is less expensive and almost as accurate in identifying most underlying conditions, making it a reasonable alternative. However, CT also increases radiation exposure. Ultrasound is growing in the specificity of its use for both diagnosis and guiding therapy.

TABLE 10.2

Indications for MRI or CT in patients with back pain

- Major trauma
- Age > 50 years
- History of cancer
- Unexplained weight loss
- Fever
- Immunosuppression
- Saddle anesthesia*
- Bowel or bladder incontinence
- Severe or progressive neurological deficit

*A physical symptom of numbness in the area of the buttocks and upper inner thighs, consistent with the portion of the body that would come into contact with a saddle.

Preventive treatment

Exercise. A systematic review of randomized controlled trials (RCTs) has found that exercise and physical activity are of moderate utility for the prevention of chronic back pain.

Lumbar supports and back schools. There is strong evidence from RCTs that lumbar supports and back schools are not effective pre-emptive interventions. A back school is a structured educational program, usually in a group setting, designed to inform patients about low back problems.

Smoking and weight reduction. Smoking and excess weight are predictors of back pain. Although there is no persuasive evidence that modifying these risk factors relieves pain, most experts who take a comprehensive disease management and rehabilitation approach to back pain advise and prescribe weight reduction to reduce mechanical load on the spine combined with exercise and cognitive behavioral therapy (CBT).

Non-pharmacological treatment

Exercise. As with the findings for acute back pain, in which a return to usual activity is the most effective therapy, meta-analyses of RCTs have shown that exercise programs reduce pain and improve function in patients with subacute, chronic or persistent postsurgical low back pain. Supervised stretching and strengthening fitness programs achieve the largest improvement compared with unsupervised exercise. One RCT has found that lumbar flexion in the early morning (i.e. a form of self-care) reduces pain intensity and costs associated with chronic non-specific low back pain.

Massage and spinal manipulation. A meta-analysis of trials that evaluated massage has concluded that the technique is beneficial for subacute and chronic back pain. Methodological flaws in the analysed trials (lack of randomization or blinding) weaken the findings. Systematic reviews and a large RCT of 1334 participants have concluded that spinal manipulation produces a small to moderate benefit at 3 months; however, its effectiveness decreases over time and at 12 months the benefit is only small.

A separate meta-analysis concluded that spinal manipulation does not reduce neck pain; moreover, case reports have documented rare but serious cerebrovascular events due to arterial damage induced by cervical manipulation.

Acupuncture. A recent meta-analysis has indicated that acupuncture produces both short-term (6 weeks) and long-term (6 months) relief of chronic back pain even when sham acupuncture is used as a comparator. However, the available data are insufficient to compare the effectiveness of acupuncture with pharmacotherapy or non-drug therapies. Acupuncture is generally safe when compared with pharmacotherapy and other procedures.

Cognitive behavioral therapy. A meta-analysis of RCTs has indicated that cognitive therapy reduces both pain intensity and behavioral expression of pain in patients with chronic pain (including those with back pain).

Other treatments. According to systematic reviews of the literature, transcutaneous electrical nerve stimulation (TENS) and the use of special corsets lack effectiveness for chronic back pain. However, they are often used as part of a comprehensive multimodal approach despite the lack of evidence to support such practice. Myofascial therapies, including trigger point needling or injections, ice, stretching and massage are routinely used to address stiffness or spasm in muscles, which are often the predominant sources of low back pain.

Pharmacological management

Non-steroidal anti-inflammatory drugs. Although non-steroidal anti-inflammatory drugs (NSAIDs) are effective for short-term symptomatic relief of acute low back pain, a systematic review found insufficient evidence to support their use for chronic low back pain.

RCTs that evaluate the combination of paracetamol (acetaminophen) plus weak opioids such as codeine or tramadol have found that these combinations reduce pain intensity. However, long-term effectiveness is unknown because of the short duration of the studies and the likelihood that tolerance would diminish the apparent analgesic benefit of such combinations during long-term clinical use.

Antidepressants. A systematic review of RCTs suggests that while antidepressants reduce the severity of chronic back pain, they do not improve functional status. As the comorbidity of depression may be quite high (15–80%) in those with chronic low back pain, particularly those treated at referral centers such as pain clinics, diagnosing depression and treating it appropriately is key to the successful treatment of back pain itself. Untreated depression reduces the positive effect of all back pain treatments.

Invasive treatment

Epidural steroid injections should not be used for non-specific low back pain; rather, their role is in the treatment of back pain that is accompanied by radicular pain. Injections can be made either translaminar via a posterior approach via the ligamentum flavum, or transforaminal via an oblique approach. Both techniques are best carried out with an image intensifier or CT control. In the acute phase of spinal nerve root irritation, early evidence points to the potential of transforaminal injection to prevent progression to chronic sciatica. However, rigorous controlled studies are not available. Of 8 patients who receive epidural steroid injections, 1 will experience at least 75% pain relief in the short term, but this benefit fades over time as only 1 out of 13 patients has 50% pain relief in the long term (12 weeks to 1 year).

Lumbar facet joint injections, medial branch blocks and radiofrequency lesioning. About 10–15% of patients with low back pain have at least part of their pain arising from the facet joints. Such patients may gain temporary relief from injection of local anesthesia and cortisone directly into the facet joint. Alternatively, the medial branch of the dorsal ramus of the appropriate spinal nerves can be blocked to provide potential temporary pain relief. This may be followed by radiofrequency lesioning to provide relief for about 6–12 months.

Such procedures do not cure back pain but may allow patients to move on to 'stretch and strengthen' programs, CBT and other options (see above).

Spinal cord stimulation (SCS) is increasingly used for the treatment of chronic back pain, particularly in patients with failed spinal surgery syndrome (persistent pain and functional limitation after spinal surgery).

A small RCT reported that patients with spinal cord stimulation were less likely to undergo reoperation. However, the value of this outcome is difficult to interpret as function and employment status were similar in both randomized groups after treatment. Recent large studies with 1-year follow-up report much better outcomes using new SCS options such as 'high frequency' and 'burst' stimulation (see Chapter 3).

Surgical treatment. Prospective cohort studies and RCTs have shown that, for patients with moderate to severe sciatica, surgical treatment yields greater short-term improvement than non-surgical treatment. On the other hand, conservative therapies should be considered the first line of treatment, as selecting a conservative treatment does not run the risk of surgical complications and the relative short-term benefit of surgery decreases over time.

There is no evidence that spinal fusion, one of the most common operations for low back problems, is superior to other surgical procedures such as laminectomy for common degenerative conditions of the spine. Interestingly, the outcome of spinal stenosis surgery does not seem to correlate with the degree of postsurgical spinal canal narrowing.

Interdisciplinary rehabilitation. Treatment designed to integrate several modalities that address the biopsychosocial factors perpetuating functional loss in chronic back pain, rather than attempting to find and treat a single cause (i.e. the 'pain generator'), is more effective for enabling patients disabled by low back pain to return to work and stay at work than are conventional or surgical treatments. Selectively combining treatments that, based on a biopsychosocial formulation, specifically address the perpetuating factor influencing recovery, appears to have the best chance of returning disabled patients to a functional quality of life.

Future treatment. Recently an 'artificial disk' has been approved for marketing, with the goal of preserving relatively normal spine architecture and mechanics after operations involving shrunken or extruded disks. Use of gene therapy such as adenovirus-mediated gene transfer to nucleus pulposus cells to halt or slow disk degeneration is also an attractive prospect.

Spinal stenosis

Spinal stenosis refers to congenital (rare) or acquired (common with advanced age) narrowing of the spinal canal or the foramina through which the nerve roots exit (Figure 10.1). Five in every 1000 people over 50 are estimated to have symptoms of spinal stenosis.

Pathophysiology. Typically, the condition occurs in the cervical or lumbar spine as a result of invasion of the spinal canal by osteophytes, tissue from hypertrophied facets, bulging disks and/or hypertrophy of the ligamentum flavum, the ligament that connects the laminae of the vertebrae and prevents excessive motion between the vertebral bodies. Compression of the medullary and lumbar cord or nerve roots produces symptoms of chronic neck or back pain along with cervical or lumbar radiculopathy, respectively.

Diagnosis. Patients with spinal stenosis experience numbness, weakness of the extremities and (for lumbar stenosis) leg pain upon walking. The last symptom, termed 'neurogenic' claudication, occurs because, when the patient walks erect, increased epidural, intrathecal and foraminal pressures compromise microcirculation to the spinal cord and nerve roots. Patients with leg pain upon walking as a result of inadequate blood flow to one or both legs are said to have 'vascular' claudication.

Symptoms of lumbar stenosis typically occur on standing or walking down stairs, and improve when the patient leans forward (e.g. on a shopping cart in a supermarket). Leaning forward (or simply

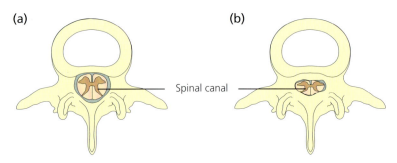

Figure 10.1 Cross-section of a vertebra with (a) a normal spinal canal and (b) stenosis of the canal and associated nerve compression.

sitting down) tends to create more space in the spinal canal and foramina, thereby decreasing compression of neural tissue and the local blood supply that feeds it.

Treatment of spinal stenosis follows the same principles as described above for back pain, with the exception of one type of spinal stenosis termed 'cauda equina syndrome', which requires immediate surgical decompression. The cauda equina is so named because the nerve roots at the caudal end of the spinal cord, which float freely within spinal fluid, resemble the tail of a horse.

Cauda equina syndrome is seen when severe pressure on the nerve fibers at the base of the spinal column results in loss of control of the bowel or bladder, pain, severe weakness, or loss of feeling in one or both legs. Immediate surgical decompression is indicated to relieve the pressure and prevent irreversible loss of spinal cord function. In addition, high-dose glucocorticoids are indicated when the cause is inoperable cancer.

> **Key points – chronic low back pain and spinal stenosis**
>
> - When the etiology of low back pain is apparent, it is most often a musculoskeletal abnormality of the lumbar spine; however, low back pain may also be referred from visceral pathology.
> - Chronic low back pain is a complex biopsychosocial process that cannot be explained on purely anatomic, biomechanical, neurophysiological, immunologic, inflammatory or neurochemical grounds.
> - Symptomatic therapy can be initiated without imaging tests in adults under 50 who lack 'red flags' – history of major trauma, cancer, or signs or symptoms of systemic disease, tumor, immunocompromise, fracture, abscess, progressive and severe neurological loss, or cauda equina syndrome.
>
> (CONTINUED)

> **Key points** *continued*
>
> - For patients over 50 and those whose findings suggest systemic disease, plain radiography and simple laboratory tests can almost completely rule out underlying systemic disease.
> - CT or MRI should be reserved for patients over 50 and those with 'red flags' (see above).
> - Exercise has moderate utility in the prevention or treatment of chronic back pain.
> - Pregabalin has small to modest analgesic efficacy.
> - Massage, spinal manipulation and acupuncture provide small-to-moderate short-term benefits.
> - There is insufficient evidence to support the long-term use of non-steroidal anti-inflammatory drugs for the treatment of chronic low back pain, particularly in light of the increased risks for gastrointestinal bleeding and cardiovascular events.
> - Epidural steroid injections produce small-to-moderate short-term pain relief.
> - Antidepressants reduce pain severity but do not improve function.
> - Integrated treatments that address the salient biopsychosocial factors perpetuating disability appear to have the best chance of returning disabled persons to a functional quality of life.
>
> See also *Fast Facts: Low Back Pain*.

Fibromyalgia

Fibromyalgia is characterized by:
- chronic widespread pain
- multiple tender points
- fatigue
- poor-quality sleep
- psychological distress and higher rates of comorbid mood disorder, in both patients and families.

The condition is more common in women, and its incidence appears to increase through middle age, after which it declines. The prevalence of fibromyalgia in the general population ranges from 0.5% to 5%, but it could be as high as 10% in women aged between 55 and 64 years. Symptoms may last for years, and relapses are common.

There is debate as to whether fibromyalgia constitutes a unique clinical entity or disease process because of the considerable overlap between patients with fibromyalgia and those with other unexplained syndromes such as irritable bowel syndrome, chronic fatigue syndrome and atypical chest pain, and because of the high association with mood disorder.

Pathophysiology. The pathophysiology of fibromyalgia remains uncertain. To date, the multidimensional (mechanical, thermal and electrical) hyperalgesia observed in patients with fibromyalgia has been explained in terms of a diffuse central sensitization leading to centrally generated symptoms and/or abnormal processing of normal sensory input. Brain-imaging studies support this explanation. Altered cytokine profiles may underlie peripheral or central sensitization.

The fatigue and sleep disturbances associated with this condition have been attributed to alterations in the hypothalamic–pituitary–adrenal (HPA) axis caused by hyperactivity of neurons that express corticotropin-releasing hormone. Cytokines have the capacity to disrupt the normal function of the HPA axis.

Diagnosis. Fibromyalgia is a clinical syndrome with no known confirmatory laboratory test. Clinical diagnosis is made on the basis of a history of widespread pain and pain triggered by digital palpation of at least 11 of 18 tender points (Figure 10.2). The pain tends to be diffuse, aching or burning, and is often described as 'head to toe'.

Pharmacological management

Non-steroidal anti-inflammatory drugs. Paracetamol (acetaminophen) and NSAIDs are commonly used to relieve pain in patients with fibromyalgia. However, RCTs have found no clear benefit of NSAIDs over placebo for this condition, which is understandable given that there is no etiologic inflammatory process associated with fibromyalgia pain. Given their potential toxicity, NSAIDs are not a cost-effective treatment option in the long term.

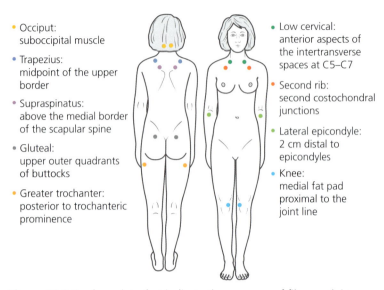

- Occiput:
  suboccipital muscle
- Trapezius:
  midpoint of the upper border
- Supraspinatus:
  above the medial border of the scapular spine
- Gluteal:
  upper outer quadrants of buttocks
- Greater trochanter:
  posterior to trochanteric prominence
- Low cervical:
  anterior aspects of the intertransverse spaces at C5–C7
- Second rib:
  second costochondral junctions
- Lateral epicondyle:
  2 cm distal to epicondyles
- Knee:
  medial fat pad proximal to the joint line

Figure 10.2 Tender points that indicate the presence of fibromyalgia.

Antidepressants. A meta-analysis of RCTs has confirmed that tricyclic antidepressants (TCAs) and serotonin–norepinephrine-reuptake inhibitors (SNRIs) such as duloxetine and milnacipran relieve stiffness, reduce tenderness and improve sleep quality in fibromyalgia. On the other hand, evidence for the effectiveness of selective serotonin-reuptake inhibitors (SSRIs) is conflicting.

Muscle relaxants. RCTs show that cyclobenzaprine, a tricyclic marketed in the USA as a muscle relaxant, is effective for fibromyalgia pain. As with all TCAs, the side-effect burden is an issue.

Weak opioids. The SNRI properties of tramadol, in addition to its weak opioid agonist activity, suggest this as a candidate for moderate fibromyalgia pain. RCTs evaluating the efficacy of tramadol and paracetamol have found that the combination of these two drugs is superior to placebo for decreasing pain intensity in fibromyalgia. However, the follow-up period was short, and the potential for tolerance and dependence has not yet been elucidated (see pages 97–8).

Anticonvulsants. The gabapentinoid pregabalin has been shown to produce small to modest benefits in patients with fibromyalgia. The results of an RCT have suggested that pregabalin reduces pain, improves sleep and reduces fatigue in patients with fibromyalgia.

Pregabalin provides pain relief in 1 in every 6 individuals, but minor adverse events also occur with the same prevalence.

Non-pharmacological treatment

Exercise. RCTs have demonstrated that aerobic exercise improves physical symptoms and anxiety scores. However, the minimal or optimal exercise regimen to produce such benefits has not yet been defined. The general approach is to combine a progressive exercise program with CBT and psychological support.

Acupuncture. There is conflicting evidence for the effectiveness of acupuncture for fibromyalgia. A systematic review of the literature could not account for the wide diversity of study results, though there is evidence of long-term benefits.

Education may include strategies for coping with symptoms, encouraging physical activity and discussion of biomedical knowledge with health providers. However, a systematic review of the efficacy of these types of program produced disappointing results as their benefits were not maintained at follow-up.

Prognosis. With appropriate treatment, mild to moderate fibromyalgia is not necessarily physically debilitating. The condition does not reduce life span.

Key points – fibromyalgia

- Fibromyalgia is characterized by chronic widespread pain, tender points, fatigue and poor sleep quality.
- Whether fibromyalgia constitutes a unique disease process is debated.
- Fibromyalgia is a clinical syndrome; there is no laboratory test that confirms the diagnosis.
- Exercise, cognitive behavioral therapy, tricyclic antidepressants (TCAs), pregabalin, serotonin–norepinephrine-reuptake inhibitors and cyclobenzaprine (with TCA mechanism of action) are effective treatments, best combined to suit the individual.

Pain due to osteoporosis

Osteoporosis is a systemic skeletal condition characterized by decreased bone density and weakened bone structure that leads to an increased risk of bone fracture.

The most common primary forms of bone loss are postmenopausal and age-related osteoporosis. Osteoporosis may also be secondary to a wide variety of medical problems, including hypercortisolism, hyperthyroidism, and long-term use of corticosteroids, hyperparathyroidism, alcohol abuse and immobilization.

Approximately 25% of postmenopausal women have osteoporosis, and in people 60 years of age or older it is the most common risk factor for non-traumatic fractures. Osteoporosis produces chronic pain due to fractures. Vertebral fracture is the most frequent complication of osteoporosis (Figure 10.3) and is associated with high rates of chronic pain, functional decline, psychosocial dysfunction and early mortality.

Diagnosis. The earliest symptom of osteoporosis is often an episode of acute severe back pain caused by a vertebral compression fracture, or acute severe groin or thigh pain caused by a hip fracture. Diagnostic

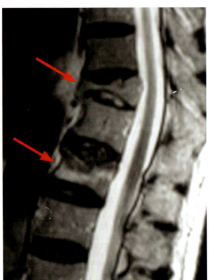

Figure 10.3 MRI scan showing two osteoporotic vertebral fractures in the thoracic region (red arrows). The lower fracture is a recent one.

work-up should include a clinical history, physical examination, laboratory evaluation, bone densitometry and radiographic imaging. This work-up will generally allow the clinician to determine the cause of osteoporosis and to institute medical interventions to slow progression or even reverse the condition.

General management. The choice of pain treatment should be tailored to the individual, as there is wide variation in the clinical presentation and the degree of physical disability associated with osteoporosis. For patients with acute or chronic pain, the treatment of pain and functional limitations should be the first priority.

Subsequent measures should include treatments aimed at maintaining bone mass to avoid new fractures, lifestyle re-education, physical therapy, physical fitness training, an appropriate course of rehabilitation to rebuild muscle mass and function, neurological and orthopedic evaluation and, for some patients, use of an orthosis.

Pharmacological management

Non-steroidal anti-inflammatory drugs are first-line treatment for mild to moderate pain secondary to a stable fracture. No trials have assessed the effect of NSAIDs on the healing of osteoporotic fractures. However, retrospective cohort studies have suggested that high doses of traditional NSAIDs could increase the likelihood of non-union after spinal fusion surgery. Conversely, RCTs that have evaluated bone healing after spinal fusion have provided no evidence that cyclooxygenase-2 (COX-2) inhibitors affect the rate of non-union at 1 year.

If pain persists, an opioid should be added. For any but the briefest of courses, opioid therapy should be approached as it is for any subacute to chronic illness. In this mostly elderly population, the approach to opioid therapy should include the initiation of a bowel regimen at the onset of therapy, consideration of breakthrough medication as needed and controlled-release formulations.

When prescribing NSAIDs or opioids, the usual cautions with respect to comorbidity (e.g. with renal or pulmonary disease, respectively) should be kept in mind.

Calcitonin is a natural hormone that exerts antiresorptive properties by blocking osteoclastic activity. The value of calcitonin treatment for postmenopausal osteoporosis remains uncertain, particularly in the prevention of fractures. However, RCTs that have evaluated calcitonin administered after fractures indicate that, given subcutaneously or intranasally, it acts as an analgesic. Pain relief occurs within 1 week of starting calcitonin. Patients also seem to have earlier mobilization than those receiving a placebo.

The mechanism of calcitonin action is not yet known. It could be mediated through an effect on nociceptive transmission or on calcitonin-binding sites in areas of the brain. Further research is required to compare the efficacy of calcitonin with standard analgesics, as 1 in every 11 individuals given calcitonin stops taking it because of adverse events such as flushing, nausea and vomiting.

Epidural analgesia. In severe acute pain refractory to systemic medications, a short-term epidural catheter may aid mobilization in patients who would otherwise be bed-bound. The catheter tip is usually placed as close as possible to the fracture, and small doses of an opioid and local anesthetic are infused. Evidence for the effectiveness of this approach is only available from case reports.

Corticosteroid injection. Similar empirical results have shown that a single epidural injection of a corticosteroid provides symptomatic relief of inflammation adjoining a new vertebral fracture. Repeated injections, however, may enhance osteoporosis and so are relatively contraindicated.

Non-pharmacological treatment

Vertebroplasty has recently been introduced for treatment of patients with osteoporosis who have acute or chronic pain following vertebral fracture. The procedure involves the injection of bone cement into the fractured vertebral body in an attempt to stabilize fractured segments and reduce pain. Case series have suggested that the procedure is associated with substantial short-term pain relief and improvements in health-related quality of life (HRQoL) that seem to persist at 6 months. Other benefits include prevention of recurrent pain, reversal of height loss and spinal deformity, and improved level of function.

In general, 1–10% of patients experience short-term complications, mainly from the extravasation of cement. These problems include increased pain and damage from pressure on the spinal cord or nerve roots, infection, bleeding and pneumothorax.

Possible long-term complications include local acceleration of bone resorption caused by the treatment itself or by a foreign-body reaction at the cement–bone interface, and increased risk of fracture in treated or adjacent vertebrae through changes in mechanical forces. Vertebroplasty has recently been evaluated in an RCT – surprisingly, there was no long-term benefit.

Kyphoplasty (sometimes referred to as balloon-assisted vertebroplasty) has been evaluated only in case series. Before injecting the cement-like material, a balloon is inserted and gently inflated inside the fractured vertebrae. Substantial pain relief has been reported during short follow-up periods.

Kyphoplasty offers a theoretical advantage over vertebroplasty as the former is believed to provide better restoration of height and better reduction of spine deformity; however, it is more expensive. To date, no head-to-head trials have compared kyphoplasty with vertebroplasty.

Key points – pain due to osteoporosis

- Osteoporosis increases the risk of bone fracture, of which vertebral fracture is the most common.
- Non-steroidal anti-inflammatory drugs are the treatment of choice for mild to moderate pain secondary to a fracture, followed by opioid therapy for more severe pain.
- In case series, vertebroplasty is associated with substantial short-term pain relief and improvements in health-related quality of life that seem to persist at 6 months.

See also *Fast Facts: Osteoporosis*.

Pain due to osteoarthritis

Osteoarthritis is a disease characterized by joint pain, distortion of joint architecture and impaired function due to articular cartilage degeneration and local inflammation. It is the most common form of arthritis and the most common cause of disability in older adults.

Osteoarthritis affects an estimated 20 million people or more in the USA and 4.5 million people in the UK. The condition is more prevalent with advancing age: people over 35 years of age have an 11% prevalence of hip osteoarthritis that increases to 36% in people over 85 years of age. Similarly, 10% of individuals over 55 years old have knee pain due to osteoarthritis; 25% of these individuals are severely disabled.

Osteoarthritis is one of the ten leading causes of disease burden in the developed world. Pain and physical limitations produced by osteoarthritis substantially affect HRQoL. Individuals with osteoarthritis have a lower HRQoL than individuals with gastrointestinal or cardiovascular conditions, or chronic respiratory diseases.

Pathophysiology. Although the causes of osteoarthritis are not completely understood, the enzymatic and mechanical breakdown of the cartilage matrix is key to the pathophysiology of the condition. Healthy cartilage is able to transmit force between the joints while maintaining almost friction-free limb movement. In osteoarthritis, these biomechanical properties are compromised; however, it is not clear whether the degeneration of cartilage precedes the onset of the disease or is a result of it.

The integrity of normal articular cartilage is maintained by a balance between anabolic and catabolic processes. This balance is disrupted in osteoarthritis. Cartilage degeneration correlates with age: senescent chondrocytes have decreased mitotic activity and are less responsive to anabolic growth factors, and thus synthesize smaller amounts of functional proteins. All of these changes lead to progressive cartilage damage and decreased capacity for regeneration.

In osteoarthritis, chondrocytes also produce an excess of nitric oxide and other inflammatory mediators such as eicosanoids and cytokines. The excessive nitric oxide produces cellular injury, inhibits cartilage synthesis and renders the chondrocyte susceptible to cytokine-induced apoptosis. In addition to promoting cartilage damage, these inflammatory phenomena predispose the patient to peripheral nerve sensitization with subsequent central sensitization and chronic pain.

Bone is also structurally abnormal in osteoarthritis. Periarticular bone has increased turnover, decreased bone mineral content and a reduced number of trabeculae, which affect its biomechanical integrity.

Diagnosis. Patients with osteoarthritis typically have morning stiffness and swelling of the involved joint (Figure 10.4), with pain that tends to worsen on weight bearing or activity, but improves with rest.

(a)

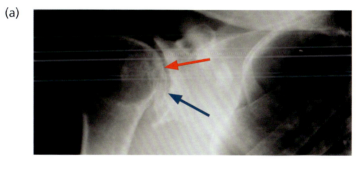

(b)

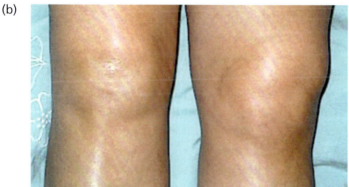

Figure 10.4 (a) Radiograph of a 65-year-old man with osteoarthritis of the shoulder. There is a marked decrease in the glenohumeral joint space (blue arrow), along with bony sclerosis (red arrow). (b) Osteoarthritis of both knees in a 67-year-old woman, with deformities and mild edema in the left knee.

Physical examination often reveals tenderness on palpation, bony enlargement, crepitus with movement and/or limitation of joint motion. Unlike in rheumatoid arthritis and other inflammatory arthritides, the inflammation in osteoarthritis, if obvious at all, is usually mild and localized to the affected joint.

General management. The goals of treatment for osteoarthritis are:
- pain relief
- prevention of complications such as muscle atrophy or deformities
- maintenance and/or improvement of functional status and HRQoL.

Treatment strategies consist of pharmacological and non-pharmacological modalities and invasive procedures.

Pharmacological management
Non-steroidal anti-inflammatory drugs. Meta-analyses have shown that NSAIDs are effective for pain relief in osteoarthritis: 59–82% of patients receiving NSAIDs report at least 50% pain relief. Paracetamol (acetaminophen) is less effective: only 20–40% of patients who receive paracetamol report pain relief of 50% or more.

Conventional NSAIDs inhibit both of the COX isoforms, COX-1 and COX-2, but COX-2 inhibitors are much more selective against the COX-2 isoform. The COX-1 isoform is produced constitutively (i.e. always produced), and it is present mainly in the gastric mucosa. COX-2 is inducible and is responsible for the enhanced formation of prostaglandins during inflammation.

Multiple RCTs have confirmed the effectiveness of COX-2 inhibitors for osteoarthritis. The major clinical interest of these selective COX-2 inhibitors has been the lower incidence of gastrointestinal bleeding than that associated with traditional NSAIDs; however, this benefit is not always present, decreases over time and falls with the concomitant use of acetylsalicylic acid (ASA; aspirin) for cardiovascular protection.

A comprehensive study of the cost-effectiveness of COX-2 inhibitors and traditional NSAIDs has found that money saved from the risk reduction of gastrointestinal adverse effects associated with COX-2 inhibitors does not offset the higher costs of these drugs during management of average-risk patients with chronic arthritis.

In addition, growing concern regarding an increase in cardiovascular events in patients receiving COX-2 inhibitors led to the withdrawal of rofecoxib and valdecoxib from the market in the USA and re-evaluation of their status in Europe. Following a thorough review in the USA and Australia, celecoxib remains on the market because of its favorable gastrointestinal safety profile.

While the efficacy and safety of NSAIDs and COX-2 inhibitors for long-term use are being re-evaluated, it seems most prudent to employ long-established NSAIDs for pain relief after careful patient selection and with ongoing monitoring. Patients receiving long-term treatment with either NSAIDs or COX-2 inhibitors should be informed that all drugs in these classes (except for ASA) carry cardiovascular risks with chronic use.

Combination therapy. The combination of NSAIDs and weak opioids (e.g. paracetamol with codeine or tramadol) seems to provide slightly greater analgesia than paracetamol alone in patients with osteoarthritis, as double-blind RCTs have shown.

Strong opioids. Given alone or in combination with NSAIDs or paracetamol, strong opioids are effective for controlling chronic arthritis pain. However, as discussed in Chapter 3, the risks must be monitored and, given the risk of death from overdose at higher doses and in combination with sedatives and anxiolytics, dose escalations should be considered carefully.

Glucosamine is a widely used therapy, but its effectiveness is unproven.

Tricyclic antidepressants. Meta-analyses of RCTs have confirmed that TCAs are effective for the treatment of osteoarthritic pain.

Capsaicin. A systematic review of published RCTs found that capsaicin decreased osteoarthritic pain (see page 101 for a general description of capsaicin).

Intra-articular therapy. When patients do not respond to a program of non-pharmacological therapy (see below) and analgesics, intra-articular injections of sodium hyaluronate or corticosteroids produce symptomatic benefit that may last for as long as 6 months. However, limited data are available on the effectiveness of multiple courses of intra-articular therapy.

Surgery. Total joint replacement, such as total hip and total knee arthroplasties, are extremely effective in improving dimensions of HRQoL. Logic and evidence indicate that the timing of surgery should be individualized on the basis of response to less invasive options and with orthopedic specialist consultation.

Indications for joint replacement include radiographic evidence of joint damage and/or moderate to severe persistent pain or disability that are not substantially relieved by an extended course of non-surgical management.

Non-pharmacological treatment

Exercise and weight loss. Exercise reduces pain and disability in patients with osteoarthritis of the hip or knee. These findings are supported by systematic reviews of the literature and a meta-analysis of RCTs on the effect of exercise on osteoarthritic pain.

Consistently, RCTs show that overweight patients with hip or knee osteoarthritis who lose weight have improved symptoms and function.

Education. A systematic review of published RCTs and non-randomized trials has suggested a beneficial effect of educational programs such as relaxation training, biofeedback, problem-solving strategies, social support or stress reduction for patients with osteoarthritis. These programs have been shown to reduce joint pain and the frequency of arthritis-related physician visits, increase physical activity and improve quality of life.

Acupuncture. The role of acupuncture for the treatment of osteoarthritis is not clear. RCTs have shown that acupuncture is not superior to sham-needling in reducing osteoarthritic pain. This equivalence implies that sham-needling has similar specific effects as acupuncture or that both methods produce substantial non-specific effects.

In the future, efforts to prevent the development or progression of osteoarthritis will probably include strategies that delay the onset of chondrocyte senescence or that replace senescent cells. These objectives can be met by disease-modifying drugs aimed at inhibiting the breakdown of cartilage or at stimulating repair activity by chondrocytes.

> **Key points – pain due to osteoarthritis**
>
> - Osteoarthritis is characterized by joint pain with loss of joint architecture and function due to articular cartilage degeneration and local inflammation.
> - Pain and limitation of physical function substantially affect health-related quality of life (HRQoL).
> - The goal of treatment is to relieve pain, prevent complications and maintain and/or improve functional status and HRQoL.
> - Exercise and weight loss are beneficial.
> - Non-steroidal anti-inflammatory drugs (NSAIDs) are effective for pain relief.
> - Ongoing concerns regarding the safety and cost-effectiveness of chronic therapy with cyclooxygenase (COX)-2 inhibitors has led to worldwide caution over their use.
> - Patients treated long term with NSAIDs or COX-2 inhibitors should be informed that all drugs in these classes (except acetylsalicylic acid [ASA]; aspirin) carry cardiovascular risks with chronic use.
> - Total joint arthroplasties are effective for improving HRQoL.
>
> See also *Fast Facts: Osteoarthritis*.

Pain due to rheumatoid arthritis

Rheumatoid arthritis is a chronic systemic autoimmune disorder characterized by joint pain and inflammation that may progress to joint destruction. Rheumatoid arthritis is the most common inflammatory arthritis and a major cause of disability; 1–2% of the world's population is affected by the condition.

Pathophysiology. A multistage theory that integrates various genetic hypotheses has been postulated. Some believe that rheumatoid arthritis originates from a bacterial or viral infection. Bacterial and viral antigenic particles have been detected in synovial tissue, and could be responsible for the initial activation of the inflammation. B cell activation and generation of autoantibodies directed to the Fc ('fragment that crystallizes') portion of human immunoglobulin G class molecules ('rheumatoid factors') could also be responsible for activation of innate immunity. The production of cytokines such as tumor necrosis factor-α and interleukin-1 by macrophages and fibroblasts in the joint, and the local expression of adhesion molecules following immune activation, promote the ingress of immune cells and the accumulation of T cells and B cells in the inflamed synovium. Cytokines and locally expressed degradative enzymes such as metalloproteinases digest the cartilage matrix and destroy articular and bone structures, resulting in pain.

Diagnosis of rheumatoid arthritis requires the presence of four or more of the criteria shown in Table 10.3. Subluxation of the atlantoaxial or cricoarytenoid joints may not be apparent, but patients with cervical spine instability are at risk of impingement of the spinal cord during routine procedures such as endotracheal intubation, and should therefore undergo neurological evaluation before any surgical intervention. Hoarseness or pain on talking should alert the clinician to possible problems with the cricoarytenoid joint.

TABLE 10.3

Criteria for diagnosis of rheumatoid arthritis

Diagnose if ≥ 4 of the following features are present
- Morning stiffness in and around joints for ≥ 1 hour before maximal improvement*
- Soft tissue swelling of ≥ 3 joint areas*
- Swelling of the proximal interphalangeal, metacarpophalangeal or wrist joints*
- Symmetric swelling*
- Subcutaneous rheumatoid nodules
- Circulating rheumatoid factor
- Radiographic erosions and/or periarticular osteopenia in hand and/or wrist joints (Figure 10.5)

*Must have been present for at least 6 weeks.

Musculoskeletal pain

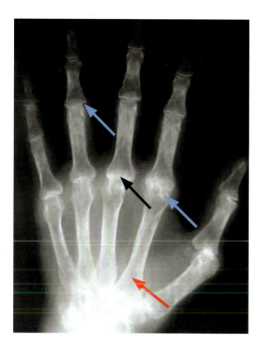

Figure 10.5 Radiograph of the hand of a 48-year-old woman with rheumatoid arthritis, showing diffuse osteopenia (red arrow), decreased interphalangeal joint spaces without sclerosis (black arrow) and subchondral cysts (blue arrows). Similar changes are observed in the carpal joints.

Pharmacological management

Non-steroidal anti-inflammatory drugs. Pharmacotherapy for rheumatoid arthritis follows a 'pyramid model' in which the first level of treatment is NSAID therapy. Meta-analysis of RCTs has confirmed that NSAIDs are effective in decreasing pain and the number of tender joints, and improving function in rheumatoid arthritis.

COX-2 inhibitors and traditional NSAIDs have similar analgesic efficacy. However, COX-2 inhibitors should not be considered as first-line treatment (see pages 156–7 for the supporting arguments).

NSAID–opioid combinations. The combination of NSAIDs and weak opioids is commonly used to produce greater analgesia than can be achieved by each individual drug.

Slow-acting antirheumatic drugs (SAARDs) are used to replace or supplement NSAIDs when the latter do not provide adequate pain control. SAARDs are distinguished from NSAIDs primarily by their assumed disease-modifying potential and delayed onset of action. Agents falling within this therapeutic class include hydroxychloroquine, gold, D-penicillamine, methotrexate, azathioprine and sulfasalazine. In much of the literature this class is also termed 'disease-modifying antirheumatic drugs' (DMARDs).

Systematic reviews of RCTs that have evaluated SAARDs have confirmed their effectiveness in reducing pain intensity and decreasing the number of painful and swollen joints. However, their use is associated with a high discontinuation rate due to adverse events, especially for azathioprine and cyclophosphamide.

Oral corticosteroids decrease joint tenderness and pain, and improve grip strength with an efficacy nearly equivalent to second-line agents previously examined in meta-analyses. The morbidity associated with chronic corticosteroid use mandates great caution in their use.

One RCT has suggested that SAARDs produce their greatest benefit when introduced early in the course of the disease.

Biological response modifiers (BRMs) are a third line of treatment based on pathogenic mechanisms. BRMs are DMARD treatments aimed at blocking the specific biological effects of inflammatory cytokines, tumor necrosis factor and other modulators of inflammation.

RCTs have indicated that BRMs are more efficacious than traditional agents because, in addition to addressing symptoms, they attenuate synovial inflammation, halt the progression of joint damage and joint destruction, and reduce disease activity in patients with long-standing rheumatoid arthritis. One-quarter of individuals treated with BRMs obtain substantial pain relief. However, the side effects may be serious, and include severe infection, increased risk of tuberculosis, lymphomas and demyelinating disease.

Tricyclic antidepressants. RCTs have consistently shown that antidepressants are efficacious for pain associated with rheumatoid arthritis and therefore should be an early part of the treatment armamentarium , although the usual cautions regarding their use apply (see page 96).

Non-pharmacological treatment

Education and behavioral therapies. A systematic review of the literature has concluded that patient education is effective in reducing pain and improving function in rheumatoid arthritis. The programs reviewed included relaxation training, biofeedback, problem-solving strategies, social support and stress reduction. Comparing its relative effectiveness with that of modalities such as NSAIDs, education gives 20–30% greater benefit overall; education is also 40% better than NSAIDs at improving functional ability and 60–80% better at reducing tender joint counts.

A systematic review of RCTs that have evaluated the effect of relaxation, biofeedback and cognitive behavioral therapies suggests that each of these therapies is an effective adjunctive treatment.

Occupational therapy improves functional ability in patients with rheumatoid arthritis, according to the results of a systematic review of RCTs.

Exercise. A meta-analysis of RCTs has shown that exercise in patients with well-controlled disease increases aerobic capacity, joint mobility and muscle strength.

Acupuncture has not been found to be of use for the treatment of pain associated with rheumatoid arthritis.

Key points – pain due to rheumatoid arthritis

- Rheumatoid arthritis is a chronic systemic autoimmune disorder characterized by joint inflammation, joint destruction and pain.
- Education, occupational therapy, exercise, relaxation, biofeedback and cognitive behavioral therapies are effective interventions.
- Pharmacological treatment follows a pyramidal model: it begins with non-steroidal anti-inflammatory drugs, is followed by slow-acting antirheumatic drugs and ends with biological response modifiers.
- Joint replacement is appropriate for the restoration of function in joints deformed by advanced rheumatoid arthritis, but intubation for anesthesia must be approached cautiously in light of potential unappreciated cricoarytenoid or atlantoaxial joint subluxation.

See also *Fast Facts: Rheumatoid Arthritis*.

Key references

American Geriatrics Society. Pharmacological management of persistent pain in older persons. *Pain Med* 2009;10:1062–83.

Atlas SJ, Keller RB, Chang Y et al. Surgical and nonsurgical management of sciatica secondary to a lumbar disc herniation: five-year outcomes from the Maine Lumbar Spine Study. *Spine (Phila Pa 1976)* 2001;26:1179–87.

Cepeda MS, Camargo F, Zea C, Valencia L. Tramadol for osteoarthritis. *Cochrane Database Syst Rev* 2006;3:CD005522.

Crawford C, Boyd C, Paat CF et al. The impact of massage therapy on function in pain populations – a systematic review and meta-analysis of randomized controlled trials: part I, patients experiencing pain in the general population. *Pain Med* 2016;17:1353–75.

Global Burden of Disease Study 2013 Collaborators. Global, regional, and national incidence, prevalence, and years lived with disability for 301 acute and chronic diseases and injuries in 188 countries, 1990–2013: a systematic analysis for the Global Burden of Disease Study 2013. *Lancet* 2015;386:743–800.

Harden RN, Song S, Fasen J et al. Home-based aerobic conditioning for management of symptoms of fibromyalgia: a pilot study. *Pain Med* 2012;13:835–42.

Hayden JA, van Tulder MW, Tomlinson G. Systematic review: strategies for using exercise therapy to improve outcomes in chronic low back pain. *Ann Intern Med* 2005;142:776–85.

Jarvik JG, Hollingworth W, Martin B et al. Rapid MRI vs radiographs for patients with low back pain: a randomized controlled trial. *JAMA* 2003;289:2810–18.

Linton SJ, van Tulder MW. Preventive interventions for back and neck pain problems: what is the evidence? *Spine (Phila Pa 1976)* 2001;26:778–87.

Manheimer E, White A, Berman B et al. Meta-analysis: acupuncture for low back pain. *Ann Intern Med* 2005;142:651–63.

Messier SP, Loeser RF, Miller GD et al. Exercise and dietary weight loss in overweight and obese older adults with knee osteoarthritis: the Arthritis, Diet, and Activity Promotion Trial. *Arthritis Rheum* 2004;50:1501–10.

Peul WC, van Houwelingen HC, van den Hout WB et al. Surgery versus prolonged conservative treatment for sciatica. *N Engl J Med* 2007;356:2245–56.

Qaseem A, Wilt TJ, McLean RM, Forciea MA; Clinical Guidelines Committee of the American College of Physicians. Noninvasive treatments for acute, subacute, and chronic low back pain: a clinical practice guideline from the American College of Physicians *Ann Intern Med* 2017;166:514–30.

Reid MC, Bennett DA, Chen WG et al. Improving the pharmacologic management of pain in older adults: identifying the research gaps and methods to address them. *Pain Med* 2011;12:1336–57.

Salerno SM, Browning R, Jackson JL. The effect of antidepressant treatment on chronic back pain: a meta-analysis. *Arch Intern Med* 2002;162:19–24.

Spiegel BM, Targownik L, Dulai GS, Gralnek IM. The cost-effectiveness of cyclooxygenase-2 selective inhibitors in the management of chronic arthritis. *Ann Intern Med* 2003;138:795–806.

Weiner DK, Marcum Z, Rodriguez E. Deconstructing chronic low back pain in older adults: summary recommendations. *Pain Med* 2016; 17:2238–46.

11 Visceral pain

In the past, viscera were considered insensitive to pain. It is now clear that visceral pain results from the activation of sensory afferent nerves that innervate internal organs such as the stomach, kidney, gallbladder, urinary bladder, intestines or pancreas. Disorders that could trigger visceral pain include distension from impaction, tumors, ischemia, inflammation and traction on the mesentery. There are a variety of pain syndromes thought to be maintained by the persistent activation of visceral nociceptive fibers. However, there is a common pathophysiology and symptomatic management approach to all of these syndromes.

Pathophysiology

Nociceptive input from the body surface travels along somatic nerves that enter spinal roots, accounting for the clear dermatomal organization of somatic pain sensations. Nociceptive information from internal organs, which are exclusively innervated by Aδ and unmyelinated C fibers, travels via more diffusely organized sympathetic and parasympathetic afferent pathways that enter the spinal cord at the thoracic and lumbar levels. In addition, visceral afferent fibers contain a greater percentage of neuroexcitatory transmitters such as substance P than do somatic afferent fibers. These differences between somatic and visceral innervation explain why sensations arising from visceral stimulation are generally more diffuse, more difficult to localize and more unpleasant than somatic sensations, and also why they are referred to poorly localized regions of the body surface (Figure 11.1). Visceral sensations are often accompanied by autonomic reflexes and symptoms such as nausea, sweating and malaise.

Three physiological classes of nociceptive viscerosensory receptors exist:
- high-threshold, which respond only to noxious mechanical stimuli
- wide-dynamic-range, which encode a wide range of innocuous and noxious stimuli
- silent, which are activated by inflammation.

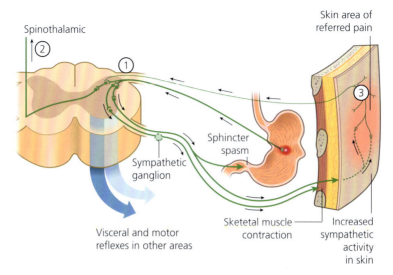

Figure 11.1 (1) Visceral and somatic nociceptive afferents converge on the same dorsal horn neuron. (2) Both visceral and somatic noxious stimuli are then conveyed, by means of the spinothalamic pathways, to the brain, where the activity is interpreted as having originated from a somatic source. (3) Referred pain is felt in the cutaneous area corresponding to the dorsal horn neurons on which the visceral afferents converged. This is accompanied by allodynia and hyperalgesia in this skin area. Also note:
- Reflex somatic motor activity results in muscle contraction, which may stimulate the parietal peritoneum and initiate somatic noxious input to the dorsal horn.
- Reflex sympathetic efferent activity may result in sphincter spasms of viscera over a wide area, causing pain remote from the original stimulus, as well as visceral ischemia and further noxious stimulation.
- Visceral nociceptors may be sensitized by norepinephrine release and microcirculatory changes.
- Increased sympathetic activity may influence cutaneous nociceptors, which may be at least partly responsible for referred pain.
- Peripheral visceral afferents branch considerably, causing much overlap in the individual dorsal roots. Only a small number of visceral afferent fibers converge on dorsal horn neurons compared with nociceptor fibers, and they converge there over a wide number of segments. Thus, dull vague visceral pain, often called deep visceral pain, is poorly localized.

High-threshold receptors exclusively innervate organs from which pain is the only conscious sensation (e.g. ureter, kidney, lungs, heart), but there are relatively few of this receptor type in organs that provide both innocuous and noxious sensations (e.g. colon, stomach, bladder).

The etiology of persistent visceral pain is often not certain. However, it is clear that visceral pain is not always linked to injury or active disease. It is believed that persistent activation of visceral fibers leads to central sensitization and to visceral hyperalgesia and that, just as for hyperalgesia from chronic somatic pain, excessive activity of N-methyl D-aspartate (NMDA) receptors is involved in this process. Autoimmune responses and inflammation could trigger the persistent activation of visceral afferent fibers. The possibility that visceral nerve injury may give rise to persistent visceral neuropathic pain is embodied in the term 'complex regional pain syndrome' (see Chapter 5).

Symptomatic management

Treatment of visceral chronic pain syndromes is aimed at symptomatic pain management. Today, visceral pain management focuses on both pharmacological and interventional techniques. Combinations of non-steroidal anti-inflammatory drugs (NSAIDs), adjuvant medications and opioids, in that sequence, form the mainstay of therapy. As stress can activate or worsen visceral pain syndromes, stress reduction techniques such as cognitive behavioral therapy (CBT) and integrative therapies can be helpful adjuncts.

When pharmacological therapies prove ineffective or are limited by side effects, regional anesthesia techniques, neurostimulation (peripheral or spinal cord) or neurosurgical techniques are considered. However, the effectiveness of these last therapies has not been evaluated rigorously, and therefore they should only be used as a last resort.

In addition, there are specific treatment modalities that are used for the treatment of specific pain syndromes.

For illustrative purposes, this chapter discusses:
- irritable bowel syndrome (IBS)
- interstitial cystitis
- male chronic pelvic pain syndrome
- endometriosis.

Irritable bowel syndrome

As much as 20% of the adult population exhibits symptoms of IBS. This functional disorder is characterized by abdominal pain, cramping, bloating, constipation and diarrhea. It occurs more often in women than in men, and it begins before the age of 35 in half of those afflicted. Most people can control their symptoms with diet, stress management and medications, but for some it can be disabling, preventing them from working, attending social events or traveling even short distances.

Diagnosis. Because IBS has no pathognomonic physical signs, its diagnosis usually requires exclusion of structural pathology with imaging or more invasive testing. It cannot be diagnosed solely from the patient's medical history. Inclusion criteria for diagnosis are shown in Table 11.1.

Treatment. Mild symptoms of IBS usually respond to stress management and changes in diet and lifestyle. If symptoms persist despite judicious use of laxatives for constipation, antidiarrheal agents or antispasmodics, tricyclic antidepressants (TCAs) may relieve pain and diarrhea, as one of their side effects is constipation.

TABLE 11.1

Criteria for the diagnosis of irritable bowel syndrome

- Abdominal pain*
- Diarrhea or constipation lasting at least 12 weeks*

Plus ≥ 2 of:

- change in the frequency of bowel movements
- change in the consistency of stool
- straining
- urgency
- a feeling of incomplete bowel movement or bloating
- mucus in the stool

*Do not have to occur consecutively.
See also *Fast Facts: Irritable Bowel Syndrome*.

As the autonomic nervous system and its enteric compartment play an important role in regulating motility and visceral perception, neurotransmitters (particularly serotonin) are targets for novel pharmacotherapeutic agents for this syndrome. Specific medications for IBS include tegaserod, a partially selective serotonin agonist (not available in the UK).

Interstitial cystitis

Interstitial cystitis is a heterogeneous chronic pain syndrome that most commonly affects women (90%). Symptoms include pain on bladder filling, pelvic pain and urinary urgency and frequency. The symptoms are often exacerbated by ovulation and during periods of stress. Two types of interstitial cystitis have been identified:
- ulcerative with bladder lesions, which responds better to therapies targeted at the bladder
- non-ulcerative, with unremarkable biopsy.

Mechanisms appear to involve both peripheral and central sensitization and inflammatory processes.

Diagnosis. In the absence of practical clinical criteria for the diagnosis of interstitial cystitis, the US National Institute of Diabetes and Digestive and Kidney Diseases of the National Institutes of Health developed criteria for research purposes. These criteria were never meant to be a gold standard for diagnosis, but they are often used as such. To be diagnosed with interstitial cystitis for research purposes, patients must have glomerulations or Hunner's ulcer on cystoscopic examination, and either bladder pain or urinary urgency in the absence of other diseases that could cause the symptoms.

Treatment. Hydrodistention of the bladder, intravesical instillation therapy and transurethral resection of diseased bladder tissue have all been used to treat interstitial cystitis. However, the effectiveness of these therapies has not been rigorously evaluated.

Sequential medication trials of amitriptyline and hydroxyzine may be helpful. Tanezumab, a monoclonal antibody with an affinity for nerve growth factor (NGF), which prevents toxins interacting with nociceptive neurons in the bladder, has shown promise in reducing pain and urgency in women with interstitial cystitis, but not in men with pelvic pain. Further medication studies are needed.

Commonly used non-surgical management strategies include careful attention to diet to avoid acidic foods that might acidify the urine, and behavioral bladder training programs. Sacral nerve stimulation is reported to be effective for extremely intractable pain; however, no controlled studies are available.

Male chronic pelvic pain syndrome

The diagnosis of male chronic pelvic pain syndrome is made in men who complain of chronic pelvic pain but who have an unrevealing examination and work-up. Interstitial cystitis (see above) and male chronic pelvic pain syndrome may be the same syndrome.

Endometriosis

Endometriosis is a common gynecologic condition that produces cyclical pain. Women complain of severe dysmenorrhea, focal pelvic tenderness and dyspareunia. The pain arises because of the dissemination of endometrium to ectopic sites during retrograde menstruation or surgery, and the subsequent establishment of deposits of ectopic endometrial tissue. In many women, endometriosis is a self-limiting disease; however, in others the biological behavior is much more unpredictable.

Diagnosis is made by laparoscopy.

Treatment of endometriosis includes therapies such as medroxyprogesterone acetate, danazol, nafarelin and gonadotropin-releasing hormone analogs. Medical therapy after surgical treatment reduces pain substantially, but trials have shown no difference postoperatively at 6 months if medical therapy is used or not. Although the efficacy of a variety of treatments has been demonstrated in randomized controlled trials, only 40–70% of women with severe cases of endometriosis become pain free.

Key points – visceral pain

- Visceral pain results from activation of sensory afferent nerves that innervate the stomach, kidney, gallbladder, urinary bladder, intestines, pancreas and other visceral organs.
- Sensations arising from visceral stimulation are generally more diffuse, more difficult to localize and more unpleasant than those associated with somatic pain.
- Visceral pain is more likely than somatic pain to be associated with autonomic signs such as pallor and sweating, or symptoms such as nausea.
- Pain syndromes such as male chronic pelvic pain syndrome, interstitial cystitis, endometriosis and irritable bowel syndrome are thought to be maintained by the persistent activation of visceral fibers, and central sensitization.
- Management includes identifying and avoiding factors that aggravate the underlying condition and individual clinical trials of medication. Neuromodulatory techniques have been reported as helpful in selected cases.

Key references

Al-Chaer ED, Traub RJ. Biological basis of visceral pain: recent developments. *Pain* 2002;96:221–5.

Austin PD, Henderson SE. Biopsychosocial assessment criteria for functional chronic visceral pain: a pilot review of concept and practice. *Pain Med* 2011;12:552–64.

Batstone GR, Doble A. Chronic prostatitis. *Curr Opin Urol* 2003;13:23–9.

Giamberardino MA. Visceral pain. *Pain: Clinical Updates* 2005;XIII: 1–6. www.iasp-pain.org

Howard FM. An evidence-based medicine approach to the treatment of endometriosis-associated chronic pelvic pain: placebo-controlled studies. *J Am Assoc Gynecol Laparosc* 2000;7:477–88.

Kapural L, Nagem H, Tlucek H, Sessler DI. Spinal cord stimulation for chronic visceral abdominal pain. *Pain Med* 2010;11:347–55.

Kream RM, Carr DB. Interstitial cystitis: a complex visceral pain syndrome. *Pain Forum* 1999;8: 139–45.

Nickel JC, Mills IW, Crook TJ et al. Tanezumab reduces pain in women with interstitial cystitis/bladder pain syndrome and patients with nonurological associated somatic syndromes. *J Urol* 2016;195:942–8.

Peeker R, Fall M. Treatment guidelines for classic and non-ulcer interstitial cystitis. *Int Urogynecol J Pelvic Floor Dysfunct* 2000;11: 23–32.

Prentice A, Deary AJ, Goldbeck-Wood S et al. Gonadotrophin-releasing hormone analogues for pain associated with endometriosis. *Cochrane Database Syst Rev* 2000;2:CD000346.

Strigo IA, Bushnell MC, Boivin M, Duncan GH. Psychophysical analysis of visceral and cutaneous pain in human subjects. *Pain* 2002;97: 235–46.

Wesselmann U, Czakanski PP. Pelvic pain: a chronic visceral pain syndrome. *Curr Pain Headache Rep* 2001;5:13–9.

12 Headache

Headache is a common complaint in the general population and one of the most common reasons people seek care from primary care providers.

Classification

Acute headache. The immediate, important first step in assessing a new headache is determining whether the headache is a serious, potentially life-threatening medical event requiring emergency evaluation and management. All the possibilities highlighted in Table 12.1 must be entertained and discarded before considering the headache to be caused by a chronic headache condition. Brain imaging, including neurovascular studies, may be needed as well as cerebrospinal fluid (CSF) pressure measurement and analysis and further evaluation by a neurologist.

TABLE 12.1
Examples of circumstances requiring emergency evaluation and management

- Acute severe head pain with neurological symptoms in an adult with no prior history of headache may indicate a cerebral vascular accident, including bleeding aneurysm
- Headache and severe eye pain suggests possible acute glaucoma
- Co-occurrence of fever associated with pneumonia or other infection with stiff neck and other neurological signs may indicate meningitis or encephalitis
- Past history of cancer suggests the possibility of intracerebral tumor
- Recent head trauma or rapid acceleration/deceleration injury suggests the possibility of intracranial bleed
- History of head/neck trauma (or diagnostic lumbar puncture) followed by severe generalized headache markedly increased by upright postures suggests tear of dura or dural cuff causing leak of cerebrospinal fluid (CSF) and low CSF pressure

Chronic headache

Assessment. As with all chronic pain, headache must be assessed systematically and classified according to its likely origin as well as its temporal pattern, aggravating and ameliorating factors and perpetuating factors and comorbidities. The headache diagnoses in Table 12.2 should be considered.

History. The history should note, as for any other pain, a general medical history, including a detailed pain history (Table 12.3). It is important to note whether the headache corresponds to any cycles (menstruation, weekends, circadian) or particular exposures (fumes, smoke, foods, etc).

TABLE 12.2
Possible diagnoses for chronic headache

- Migraine: usually unilateral throbbing and episodic; often (~ 25%) preceded by aura; associated with sensory phobia to light, noise and movement
- Tension-type: usually band-like pain that is generally steady; often starts in occipital region
- Cluster: very intense and disabling; lasts for days to weeks at a time
- Sinus: with facial frontal pain, often associated with fever or allergies
- Occipital neuralgia and cervicogenic headache associated with cervical spine pathology
- Traumatic brain injury: can have multiple presentations in the context of a history of motor vehicle accidents, head trauma from falls or sports, or exposure to blast waves
- Mass lesion: from primary or secondary tumor, abscess or chronic subdural hematoma
- Transform headache: caused by frequent regular use of short-acting analgesics of any class (medication 'rebound' effects)
- Trigeminal neuralgia may sometimes present as headache (see Chapter 4)

TABLE 12.3

Diagnostic indicators that can be obtained from a careful history

Headache type	Location	Precipitants
Tension	Often bilateral. Starts in occipital region	Stress, postural factors, injury, cervical spine disease
Migraine	Usually unilateral. Temples	Triggers in order of decreasing frequency: • stress (~ 75%) • menstruation • not eating • weather changes • sleep loss • odors • neck pain • bright lights • alcohol • smoke • food • heat • exercise (~ 20%)
Cluster	Usually unilateral (side may change in 15%)	Seasonal for some
Chronic paroxysmal hemicrania (CPH)	Ocular, frontal, temporal and adjacent areas	Sometimes neck movement
Sinus	Facial	Upper respiratory tract infection, allergies
Transform (rebound)		Regular, frequent dosing of short-acting medication
Occipital neuralgia	Occipital region, often starting in neck	Position of neck
Myofascial	Neck, occipital region	Position, spine pathology
Traumatic brain injury	Variable	History of trauma, sports, concussion

Pattern/progression	Duration	Frequency
Progressing to band-like headache	Hours, days (rarely)	Episodic
68% have prodrome of nausea, vomiting, visual or mood symptoms Progresses to throbbing headache that is usually unilateral and often disabling, with sensory sensitization	Hours, sometimes days	Episodic
Lacrimation, nasal stuffiness, photophobia	Several days	Once or several times yearly
Modified 'cluster pattern' Complete relief with indometacin (indomethacin)		Episodic
Sometimes fever, tender over sinuses		Episodic
	Chronic, daily	Chronic, daily
Can progress to migraine-type headache	Variable	Variable
	Variable	Variable
Can be refractory to treatment	Variable, can be constant	Variable, can be daily with migraine-type flares

As emotional factors often trigger tension or migraine headache, psychosocial assessment for the relationship of stressful events to headache onset and extant stressors or psychiatric comorbidities will be important for risk management and treatment planning. Diagnostic testing, particularly brain imaging, may be appropriate.

Pathophysiology and associated signs and symptoms

Recent literature has tended to blur what were once thought to be clear distinctions between headaches without a clear anatomic generator, such as tension headache compared with migraine headache. However, it is useful to consider migraine headache and tension headache differently for therapeutic reasons.

Migraine headache is now thought to be a condition in which there is cortical neuronal hyperexcitability and/or brainstem dysfunction which activates peripheral nociceptors of the trigeminal neurovascular system. An increase in excitatory neurotransmitters such as glutamate and reduced intracortical inhibition are associated with meningeal inflammation and peripheral sensitization leading to dilation of cerebral vessels and pain. Further activation of the trigeminal nucleus leads to the characteristic signs of central sensitization usually associated with the clinical picture of full-blown migraine, during which almost any sensory stimulus will worsen the headache. These signs and symptoms include allodynia over the face and head, photophobia and sensitivity to noise or movement, causing patients to want to lie down in a dark, completely quiet room until the headache passes. There appears to be a genetic predisposition to migraine in some patients.

Tension headache, thought to be due to myofascial pain in the muscles of the head and neck, may be activated by stress and postural factors, or by neural stimuli from an old injury and/or cervical spine disease. These headaches can themselves activate a migraine headache in some patients.

Transform headache, often called rebound headache, is caused when the pain-suppressing effects of a short-acting sedative, anxiolytic and/ or analgesic wear off so that the manifestations of the sensitized state of the central nervous system (CNS) resumes, often leading to daily headache. Hence caution against the regular, daily or almost daily use of these drugs for headache control is advised.

Sinus headache is caused by allergy- or infection-induced sinus inflammation with subsequent blockage and increased pressure.

Psychological processes. Stress is the most common trigger of both migraine (~75%) and tension headache, and like all persistent or recurrent pain, the headaches themselves and their effects on function and quality of life can be stressful to patients, their families and their associates. As with all pain syndromes, the cycle of pain–stress–pain–dysfunction–stress–pain etc. in headache should be identified, and treatments targeted to each of the predisposing, precipitating and perpetuating factors to whatever degree is possible.

Physical examination

While many common headaches can be diagnosed by history alone, to rule out dangerous causes, physical examination of the head and neck and cranial nerves as well as physiological parameters such as vital signs (e.g. fever) and mental status (with particular attention being paid to neurological function) is necessary. For example, palpation over the occipital nerve can precipitate the pain of occipital neuralgia and trigger points in the neck and trapezius can radiate rostrally causing headache. Palpation of a very prominent and sensitive superficial temporal artery can point to a possible diagnosis of temporal arteritis; this is a crucial diagnosis because if left untreated blindness is a likely complication.

Signs and symptoms of cervical spine pathology, such as tenderness over upper cervical facet joints may point to a need for imaging of the cervical spine and possible diagnostic medial branch blocks; this could lead to a diagnosis of 'cervicogenic headache'. As emotional factors often trigger tension or migraine headaches, psychosocial assessment for stressors or psychiatric comorbidity is important.

Diagnostic testing, particularly brain imaging, may be appropriate to rule out intracerebral causes.

Diagnostic tests

For most chronic headaches, diagnostic tests are unnecessary except when a 'red flag' on history or physical examination indicates concern for an intracerebral mass and the need for imaging, or history and physical examination indicate a need for spinal evaluation and related imaging. In occipital neuralgia, sometimes neural blockade of the occipital nerves can help with diagnosis. Administration of indometacin (indomethacin) results in complete relief of chronic paroxysmal hemicrania (CPH) and this effect continues with long-term treatment. Cluster headache diagnosis may be aided by the autonomic features and at least partial response to inhaled oxygen.

Treatment

Migraine. The treatment approach for migraine is best conceptualized as longitudinal chronic disease management in three parts: preventive measures, abortive treatment and symptom management. This approach is based on understanding the phenomenological pattern of each individual's headache, as in Figure 12.1.

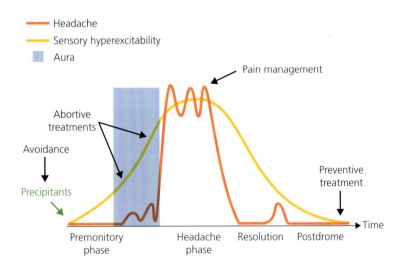

Figure 12.1 The natural course of a typical migraine attack. Adapted with permission from Linde M. *Acta Neurol Scand* 2006;114:71–83.

First, preventive treatments aim to reduce the frequency, severity and duration of attacks and include daily use of medications such as antidepressants, anticonvulsants, α_2-agonists, and β-blockers (Table 12.4).

Second, once prodromal or actual migraine symptoms occur, a stepped-care approach should be taken (Table 12.5). It is important to

---

TABLE 12.4
Preventive treatments for migraine headaches

Antidepressants
- SSRIs (e.g. sertraline, fluoxetine, citalopram)
- SNRIs (e.g. duloxetine, venlafaxine, milnacipran)
- Tricyclic antidepressants (e.g. amitriptyline)

Beta-blockers
- Propanolol

Anticonvulsants
- Valproate
- Topiramate
- Gabapentin
- Pregabalin

Others
- Verapamil

SNRI, serotonin–norepinephrine-reuptake inhibitor; SSRI, selective serotonin-reuptake inhibitor.

TABLE 12.5
Stepped-care approach to adopt for prodromal or actual migraine symptoms

- **Initial treatment:** attempt to abort progression to full-blown migraine by removing triggers, relaxation and oral NSAIDs
- **Next:** if initial treatment is not successful, oral or intramuscular or nasal triptans, which have high efficacy and are generally well tolerated; several should be tried until the most effective abortive treatment is found
- **If migraine persists:** rescue doses of analgesics and sedatives such as short-acting opioids and benzodiazepines. Inducing sleep often terminates the attack

NSAID, non-steroidal anti-inflammatory drug.

avoid frequent regular dosing (more than twice weekly) of short-acting analgesics or sedatives such as compounds containing butalbital (a short-acting barbiturate often compounded with non-steroidal anti-inflammatory drugs [NSAIDs] or paracetamol [acetaminophen]), to reduce the incidence of transform (rebound) daily headaches.

Psychotherapies, such as support/directive and cognitive behavioral therapies (CBT), may help patients manage a complex interaction of factors that perpetuate headache.

Botulinum toxin injections have been reported to be successful in some case series, but the clinical trials are equivocal; a trial should be reserved for treatment-resistant patients.

For intractable migraine and occipital neuralgia, non-invasive methods of vagal neurostimulation and transcranial magnetic neurostimulation may serve as useful adjuncts to more conventional therapies. Trials of more invasive forms of neuromodulation in the form of temporary insertion of suboccipital electrodes result in about 50% of these patients proceeding to permanent implantation of electrodes with a pulse generator.

Tension headache. Management of episodic tension-type headaches starts with understanding the precipitants of the headaches. This is best accomplished by a headache diary in which the patient records all headaches and their contexts, either in a small notebook, on headache diary sheets or in a personal digital assistant (PDA). Once precipitants are identified, intervention strategies should proceed as follows.
- For stress-induced headache, a stress management program, usually delivered in CBT, that trains the patient to avoid and/or manage precipitating stressors and to relax and stretch at onset of headache.
- For positional headache, such as that activated by poor ergonomics at a computer terminal, positional and seating changes, stretching routines and icing can be helpful.

At the onset of headache, modulation techniques are initiated, such as stretching and icing, and relaxation techniques. Usually analgesics such as NSAIDs or paracetamol suffice, although other medications such as tramadol may be tried in more severe forms. The medical custom in some countries, such as the USA, includes use of pills, combining a barbiturate, butalbital, and caffeine with paracetamol or acetylsalicylic acid (ASA; aspirin). Regular and frequent use (more than two to three times weekly) of these and other short-acting sedatives and anxiolytics as well as opioids should be avoided because of the potential for developing transform (rebound) headache, medication dependency or even addiction.

Occipital neuralgia. Pressure over occipital nerves or nerve injury due to trauma or surgery may activate headache symptoms. Nerve block may eliminate headache symptoms temporarily or for extended periods. Such blocks do not accurately predict the outcome of trial suboccipital nerve stimulation (see above).

Myofascial headache. Treatment includes awareness and avoidance of triggers, such as posture and stress. Analgesics are used with usual cautions. Trigger point injections may give short-term benefit, and physical therapy may be helpful.

Key points – headache

- In patients without history of chronic headaches, determine whether an acute new headache is a serious, potentially life-threatening condition.
- In chronic headache:
  - use a headache diary to differentiate headache type and establish pattern of triggers to enable self-management strategies
  - institute preventive measures such as trigger avoidance, stress control and medication
  - institute abortive regimen appropriate for headache type
  - migraine: non-steroidal anti-inflammatory drugs (NSAIDs), stress control, triptans
  - tension/myofascial: NSAIDs, stress control, icing, stretching
  - avoid regular frequent analgesic use to reduce incidence of transform (rebound) headache physical dependency.

Key references

Anon. The International Classification of Headache Disorders, 2nd edn. *Cephalalgia* 2004;24(suppl 1):9–160.

Ashina S, Lyngberg A, Jensen R. Headache characteristics and chronification of migraine and tension-type headache: A population-based study. *Cephalalgia* 2010;30:943–52.

Bigal ME, Ashina S, Burstein R et al. Prevalence and characteristics of allodynia in headache sufferers: a population study. *Neurology* 2008;70:1525–33.

Boardman HF, Thomas E, Millson DS, Croft PR. The natural history of headache: predictors of onset and recovery. *Cephalalgia* 2006;26:1080–8.

Francis GJ, Becker WJ, Pringsheim TM. Acute and preventive pharmacologic treatment of cluster headache. *Neurology* 2010;75:463–73.

Kindelan-Calvo P, Gil-Martínez A, Paris-Alemany A et al. Effectiveness of therapeutic patient education for adults with migraine. A systematic review and meta-analysis of randomized controlled trials. *Pain Med* 2014;15:1619–36.

Linde M. Migraine: a review and future directions for treatment. *Acta Neurol Scand* 2006;114:71–83.

Lipton RB, Silberstein SD, Saper JR et al. Why headache treatment fails. *Neurology* 2003;60:1064–70.

Loder E, Rizzoli P. Tension-type headache. *BMJ* 2008;336:88–92.

Maizels M, Burchette R. Rapid and sensitive paradigm for screening patients with headache in primary care settings. *Headache* 2003;43:441–50.

Merskey H, Bogduk N, eds. *Classification of Chronic Pain. Descriptions of Chronic Pain Syndromes and Definitions of Pain Terms*, 2nd edn. Seattle: IASP Press, 1994:77–94.

Robbins MS, Grosberg BM, Napchan U et al. Clinical and prognostic subforms of new daily-persistent headache. *Neurology* 2010;74:1358–64.

Schwedt TJ, Vargas B. Neurostimulation for treatment of migraine and cluster headache. *Pain Med* 2015;16:1827–34.

Silberstein SD, Holland S, Freitag FG et al. Evidence-based guideline update: pharmacological treatment for episodic migraine prevention in adults. *Neurology* 2012;78:1337–45.

Sillay KA, Sani S, Starr PA. Deep brain stimulation for medically intractable cluster headache. *Neurobiol Dis* 2010;38:361–8.

Smitherman TA, Burch R, Sheikh H, Loder E. The prevalence, impact, and treatment of migraine and severe headaches in the united states: a review of statistics from national surveillance studies. *Headache* 2013;53:427–36.

Acknowledgments

As clinicians and teachers we recognize the multidisciplinary and interdisciplinary nature of chronic pain and those who treat it. This book is dedicated to: our families, in grateful acknowledgment of their support during our often long hours; our colleagues, who have shared and thereby lightened our own professional burdens; and our patients and their families, who have sought to reclaim lives taken from them by chronic pain. We also thank Dan Carr and Soledad Cepeda who 'set the scene' in the first edition of this book.

Useful resources

UK
The British Pain Society
info@britishpainsociety.org
www.britishpainsociety.org

Chronic Pain Policy Coalition
www.policyconnect.org.uk/cppc

Pain Concern
info@painconcern.org.uk
www.painconcern.org.uk

The Pain Relief Foundation
administrator@painrelieffoundation.org.uk
www.painrelieffoundation.org.uk

Trigeminal Neuralgia Association UK
admin@tna.org.uk/help@tna.org.uk
www.tna.org.uk

USA
Agency for Healthcare Research and Quality
www.ahrq.gov

Alliance of State Pain Initiatives (Resource Center)
trc@mailplus.wisc.edu
www.trc.wisc.edu

American Academy of Neurology
memberservices@aan.com
www.aan.com

American Academy of Orofacial Pain
www.aaop.org

American Academy of Pain Medicine
info@painmed.org
www.painmed.org

American Chronic Pain
Association
Toll-free: 800 533 3231
ACPA@theacpa.org
https://www.theacpa.org

American Pain Society
info@americanpainsociety.org
www.americanpainsociety.org

American Society for Pain
Management Nursing
aspmn@kellencompany.com
www.aspmn.org

Facial Pain Association
info@tna-support.org
www.fpa-support.org

People in Pain Network
info@pipain.com
www.pipain.com

International
Australian Pain Society
aps@apsoc.org.au
www.apsoc.org.au

Canadian Pain Society
office@canadianpainsociety.ca
www.canadianpainsociety.ca

European Pain Federation
secretary@efic.org
www.europeanpainfederation.eu

Faculty of Pain Medicine of the
Australian and New Zealand
College of Anaesthetists
www.fpm.anzca.edu.au

International Association for the
Study of Pain
IASPdesk@iasp-pain.org
www.iasp-pain.org

FastTest

You've read the book ... now test yourself with key questions from the authors

- Go to the FastTest for this title *FREE* at fastfacts.com
- Approximate time **10 minutes**
- For best retention of the key issues, try taking the FastTest before and after reading

International Myopain Society
info@myopain.org
www.myopain.org

International Pelvic Pain Society
info@pelvicpain.org
www.pelvicpain.org

Painaustralia
lesley.brydon@painaustralia.org.au
www.painaustralia.org.au

PainSA
info@painsa.org.za
www.painsa.org.za

Trigeminal Neuralgia Association of Canada
president@tnac.org
www.tnac.org

Other useful resources
Australian and New Zealand College of Anaesthetists
Acute Pain Management: Scientific Evidence, 4th edn, 2015.
www.fpm.anzca.edu.au/documents/apmse4_2015_final

Bandolier Oxford Pain Site
www.bandolier.org.uk/booth/painpag/index2.html

National Institute for Health and Clinical Excellence
Neuropathic pain in adults: pharmacological management in non-specialist settings. Clinical guideline CG173. NICE, 2013.
www.nice.org.uk/guidance/cg173

Cousins MJ, Carr DB, Horlocker T, Bridenbaugh PO, eds. *Neural Blockade in Clinical Anesthesia & Pain Medicine*, 4th edn. Philadelphia: Wolters Kluwer/Lippincott, Williams & Wilkins, 2009.
Specifically, the following chapters:

– Binder A, Baron R. Complex regional pain syndrome including applications of neural blockade, pp1154–68.

– Burton AW, Phan PC, Cousins MJ. Treatment of cancer pain, pp1111–53.

– Carr DB, Cousins MJ. Spinal route of analgesia, pp886–947.

– Niv D, Gofeld M. Percutaneous neural destructive techniques, pp991–1035.

– Prager JP, Stanton-Hicks M. Neurostimulation, pp948–90.

– Siddall PJ, Cousins MJ. Introduction to pain mechanisms: implications for neural blockade, pp661–92.

Deer TR, Leong MS, Buvanendran A et al, eds. *Comprehensive Treatment of Chronic Pain by Medical Interventional, and Integrative Approaches. The American Academy of Pain Medicine Textbook on Patient Management.* Springer, 2013.

Index

Aβ fibers 15, 17, 18
acetaminophen 62–3, 141, 147, 156, 157, 182
acetylsalicylic acid (aspirin) 62, 86, 156
aciclovir 100
acupuncture 141, 149, 158, 163
addiction 42–4, 59
Aδ fibers 9, 166
adjective rating scale 35, 36
agomelatine 64
aldose reductase inhibitors 94–5
alendronate 65, 86
allodynia 14
  mechanisms 15, 17
  pain syndromes 92, 99, 100, 112, 120
amitriptyline 64, 95, 101, 113, 170
AMPA receptors 17
amputation 23, 117, 120–2
analgesics 25–7, 54–65
anesthesia dolorosa 76
anesthetics, intravenous 65, 114
anterior cingulate cortex 23
anticonvulsants 64
  central pain 113
  CRPS 87
  diabetic neuropathy 96–7
  fibromyalgia 148–9
  migraine 181
  phantom pain 122
  postherpetic neuralgia 101
  trigeminal neuralgia 75–6
antidepressants 63–4
  migraine 181
  musculoskeletal pain 142, 148
  neuropathic pain 86, 95–6, 113, 122
antiepileptics *see* anticonvulsants

antiviral therapy 100
anxiety 8, 26, 41, 130
ASIC receptors 9, 10
aspirin (acetylsalicylic acid) 62, 86, 156
assessment of pain 30–45, 132–3
autonomic hyperreflexia 108–9
AV411 (MN-166, ibudilast) 18
azathioprine 161–2

back pain
  cancer 128, 129
  chronic low 50–1, 137–46
  osteoporosis 150–1
  red flags 139
back schools 140
baclofen 65, 87, 116
behavioral therapies 162–3
biological response modifiers 162
bisphosphonates 63, 86
bone metastases 128, 131, 134
bone scans 44, 84, 131
botulinum toxin 102, 182
brachial plexus avulsion 114
brain
  lesions 106–7, 109–10
  neuroplastic changes 23–4
  pain pathways 9, 11
breakthrough pain 59
Brown–Séquard syndrome 114
Budapest criteria 80
buprenorphine 56, 57

calcitonin 65, 86, 152
cancer pain 126–35
  pathophysiology 127–32
  treatment 56–7, 63, 133–4
cannabinoids 18, 114

capsaicin 87, 101, 157
carbamazepine 64, 75–6, 96–7, 113
cauda equina syndrome 145
causalgia 79
celecoxib 61–2, 157
celiac plexus block 65–6
central pain 14, 106–16
central sensitization 12, 13, 17, 26
cervicogenic headache 175, 179
C fibers 9, 18, 166
character, pain 33
chemotherapy 129, 134
children 85, 99–100, 127
chronic paroxysmal hemicrania 176–7, 180
chronification, pain 25, 26, 47–51
citalopram 64
classification of pain 7
claudication 128, 144
clodronate 65
clomipramine 86
clonidine 61, 65, 89, 116
cluster headache 175, 176–7, 180
codeine 62, 141, 157
cognitive behavioral therapy (CBT) 85, 102, 113, 141, 182
complex regional pain syndrome (CRPS) 79–90
  diagnostic criteria 80, 81
  pathophysiology 14, 24, 79–84
  post-stroke 110
congenital insensitivity to pain 22
constipation 57–8
cordotomy 66–7
corticosteroids
  epidural 142, 152
  intra-articular 157
  systemic 86, 101, 162

188

Index

COX-2 inhibitors 61–2, 151, 156–7, 161
cranial nerves, evaluation 39
CRPS *see* complex regional pain syndrome
CT scan 44, 139
cyclobenzaprine 148
cyclophosphamide 162
cystitis, interstitial 170–1
cytokines 17, 19, 83, 160

danazol 171
deep brain stimulation 114
Defense and Veterans Pain Rating Scale (DVPRS) 37
depression 8, 26, 41, 130, 142
desipramine 64, 95, 113
desvenlafaxine 64
dexamethasone 65
dextromethorphan 65
diabetic neuropathy 14, 92–8, 103
diagnostic tests 44
disease-modifying antirheumatic drugs (DMARDs) 162
disk disease, degenerative 129, 138, 143
dorsal horn 9, 12, 17, 167
dorsal root entry zone (DREZ) lesioning 114–16
dorsal root ganglia 9, 11, 15–16
dorsal root ganglion stimulation 68, 89
duloxetine 64, 95, 96, 148

education 48–9, 119–20, 149, 158, 162–3
endometriosis 171
epidural analgesia 67, 89, 119, 142, 152
epilepsy 106
erythromelalgia 22
escitalopram 64
etanercept 18
examination, physical 38–41

exercise 52, 140, 149, 158, 163
extinction 23

facet joint injections 142
fentanyl 59
fibromyalgia 146–9
flecainide 65
fluoxetine 64
fractures 44, 150–1, 152–3
functional MRI 24, 27

GABA (γ-aminobutyric acid) 20
GABA agonists 65, 87, 114
gabapentin 64
  CRPS 87, 89
  diabetic neuropathy 95, 96–7
  postherpetic neuralgia 101
  trigeminal neuralgia 76
gait 39
Gasserian ganglion 73, 74
gate control theory 7–8
gene therapy 143
genetics 21–2, 118–19
glial cells 17–20
global health burden 8
glucosamine 157
gold 161–2
GTP cyclohydrolase 1 (GCH1) 21
guanethidine 87

headache 128, 129, 174–83
herpes zoster, acute 98–9, 100–1
history, pain 31–8
hyaluronate, sodium 157
hydromorphone 56
hydroxychloroquine 161–2
hydroxyzine 170
hyperalgesia 12, 54, 83, 128
visceral 168

ibudilast (AV411, MN-166) 18
imaging 27, 44, 74, 75, 106, 139

imipramine 95
indometacin 180
inflammation 15, 26, 83, 128
inhibition 11, 12
  loss of 20–1
intensity, pain 33–8
interdisciplinary care 48, 49–51, 143
interleukin (IL)-1 17, 83, 160
interleukin (IL)-6 17, 83
interstitial cystitis 170–1
intra-articular therapy 157
intraspinal drug administration (ISDA) 67, 116
invasive procedures 65–8
irritable bowel syndrome 169–70

Jannetta procedure 76
joint pain 52, 154–63

ketamine
  systemic infusion 63, 65, 89, 102, 114, 122
  transnasal 59
kyphoplasty 153

lamotrigine 64, 76, 113
lidocaine 63, 65
  regional infusion 89
  skin patches 102
  systemic infusion 76, 87, 102, 114
local anesthetics 65, 114, 142
  see also lidocaine; mexiletine
location, pain 33
lumbar stenosis 144–5
lumbar supports 140

macrophages 15, 131
magnetic resonance imaging (MRI) 44, 74, 75, 106, 139

189

magnetic resonance spectroscopy 27
male chronic pelvic pain syndrome 171
management, pain 47–70
 new developments 25–7
 passive 52–3
 pharmacotherapy 53–65
massage 140–1
mechanisms of pain 8–14
medial branch blocks 142
meditation 52
medroxyprogesterone acetate 171
memantine 65
memory and pain 22–3
mental status examination 38
meperidine 57
methadone 56, 58–9, 61, 65, 98
methotrexate 161–2
mexiletine 65, 114
microvascular decompression 76, 77
migraine 175, 176–7, 178, 179, 180–2
milnacipran 64, 95, 96, 148
minocycline 18
mirror therapy 113, 122
mirtazapine 64
MN-166 (ibudilast, AV411) 18
mood, assessment 41
morphine 55, 56, 57, 116
motor dysfunction, CRPS 82
motor system, evaluation 39
multimodal treatment 53, 112–13, 133, 141
multiple sclerosis 18, 73, 106
muscle relaxants 148
musculoskeletal examination 40–1
musculoskeletal pain 137–63
myofascial headache 176–7, 183
myofascial therapies 141

nafarelin 171
naloxone 56, 57–8
$Na_v1.7$ channels 22
$Na_v1.8$ channels 65, 93, 121
nerve injury see peripheral nerve injury
neurodestructive neurosurgery 66–7
neurokinin-1 (NK1) receptors 12, 13
neurological examination 38–9
neurolytic blocks 65–6
neuromas 16, 121
neuromodulation 67–8
neuronal reorganization 17–20
neuropathic pain 14–21
 cancer 128, 129, 131–2
 mechanisms 14–21, 23–4
 pharmacotherapy 63–5
 spinal cord injury 110, 111, 112
 types 14
neuroplasticity 8, 22–4
neurostimulation 67–8, 122
nitric oxide (NO) 12, 13, 17, 21, 154–5
NMDA receptors 12, 13, 17, 168
nociceptive pathways 9, 11
nociceptors 8–9
non-steroidal anti-inflammatory drugs (NSAIDs) 61–3
 CRPS 85
 migraine 181, 182
musculoskeletal pain 141, 147, 151, 156–7, 161
noradrenaline-reuptake inhibitors (NRIs) 64
nortriptyline 64, 95, 113
numeric rating scale (NRS) 35, 36

occipital neuralgia 175, 176–7, 179, 180, 182, 183

occupational therapy 85, 163
opioids 54–61
 advances in delivery 27
 cancer pain 132, 133
 musculoskeletal pain 141, 148, 151, 157, 161
 neuropathic pain 86, 97–8, 102, 114, 122
 withdrawal symptoms 60
osteoarthritis 154–9
osteoporosis 83, 86, 129, 150–3
oxycodone 56, 57–8
oxycontin 56

pain
 classification 7
 defining 7–8, 12
 mechanisms 8–14
pain, enjoyment and general activity (PEG) scale 35, 36
paracetamol see acetaminophen
paroxetine 64
pathophysiology, pain 14–25, 26
pelvic pain 70, 170–1
D-penicillamine 161–2
peripheral nerve injury 14–21
 CRPS 79, 81
 surgical 117, 119, 120–1
peripheral nerve stimulation (PNS) 68–70, 120
peripheral sensitization 9–12, 26
persistent postsurgical pain (PPSP) 117–23, 127, 129
phantom experiences 121–2
phantom pain 14, 121–2
pharmacogenetics 27, 54
pharmacotherapy 53–65
phentolamine 87
physical activity 52, 140, 149, 158, 163
physical dependence 59

physical therapy 85, 113
postamputation pain 23, 120–2
postherpetic neuralgia 14, 98–103
postincisional pain 14, 120
post-stroke pain 106–7, 109–10, 112–16
postsurgical pain *see* persistent postsurgical pain
potentiation 9–12
PQRSTU mnemonic 30
prednisone 65
pregabalin 64
 central pain 113
 CRPS 89
 diabetic neuropathy 95, 96, 97
 fibromyalgia 148–9
 postherpetic neuralgia 101
 trigeminal neuralgia 76
propofol 65, 114
protein kinase C (PKC) 12, 13, 17
psychological processes 84, 130, 179
psychological therapies 85, 102, 113, 182
psychosocial assessment 41–2
purine (P2X and P2Y) receptors 9, 10

quality of life 42, 43

radiation, pain 33
radiofrequency lesioning 67, 142
radionuclide therapy 134
radiotherapy 129, 134
rebound headache *see* transform headache
reboxetine 64
referred pain 167
reflex sympathetic dystrophy 79
reflex testing 39
relaxation 52, 163

respiratory depression 56–7
rheumatoid arthritis 129, 159–63
rofecoxib 61, 157

sacral nerve stimulation (SNS) 70, 171
Sativex 18
sciatica 21, 119, 138, 142, 143
SCN9A gene 22
selective serotonin-reuptake inhibitors (SSRIs) 64, 95–6
self-management 51–2
sensory perception 39
serotonin–norepinephrine-reuptake inhibitors (SNRIs) 64
migraine 181
musculoskeletal pain 148
neuropathic pain 86, 95–6, 101, 113
sertraline 64
shingles *see* herpes zoster, acute
sinus headache 175, 176–7, 179
sleep disturbances 41, 147
slow-acting antirheumatic drugs (SAARDs) 161–2
smoking 140
SNX-111 (ziconotide) 67
sodium channels 15, 16, 22, 64–5, 121
somatosensory cortex 23–4
spinal analgesic chemotherapy 67
spinal cord compression 128
spinal cord injury (SCI) 24, 106, 107–8, 110–16
spinal cord, pain pathways 9, 11, 166, 167
spinal cord stimulation (SCS) 68, 88, 102, 114, 142–3
spinal manipulation 140–1
spinal stenosis 144–6

spinal surgery 143
spine, examination 41
spinothalamic tract 11, 23, 167
splanchnic block 66
stepped care model 47–9, 133, 181
steroids *see* corticosteroids
STORM 44
stress, psychological 23, 84, 102, 179
stroke 106–7, 109–10, 112–16
stump pain 121
substance abuse 42–4, 57
suicide risk 41, 77
sulfasalazine 162
sympathectomy, surgical 88
sympathetically maintained pain 83–4
sympathetic blockade 87, 101
sympathetic fibers 15–16

tanezumab 170–1
tapentadol 60
tegaserod 170
temporal arteritis 75, 179
tender points 147, 148
tendon reflex testing 39
tension headache 175, 176–7, 178, 179, 182–3
tetrahydrocannabinol (THC) 18, 114
thalamic syndrome 109–10
total pain concept 132
toxic neuropathy 14
tramadol 59–60, 97–8, 141, 148
transcranial magnetic neurostimulation 122, 182
transcutaneous electrical nerve stimulation (TENS) 53, 102, 122, 141
transform headache 175, 176–7, 178–9
traumatic brain injury 175, 176–7

Treatment Outcomes in Pain Survey (TOPS) 42, 43
tricyclic antidepressants (TCAs) 64
  migraine 181
  musculoskeletal pain 148, 157, 162
  neuropathic pain 86, 95–6, 101, 113
trigeminal nerve 73
trigeminal neural complex, invasive procedures 76–7
trigeminal neuralgia 14, 64–5, 73–7, 175
triptans 181
TRP receptors 9, 10

tumor necrosis factor (TNF)α 17, 83, 160
vagal neurostimulation 182
valdecoxib 61, 157
valproate, sodium 64, 101, 113
variability in pain response 21–2
varicella zoster virus (VZV) 98–9
vaccination 99–100
venlafaxine 64, 95, 96
vertebral fractures 44, 150, 152–3
vertebroplasty 152–3

vibration test 94
vigabatrin 64
visceral nociceptors 166–8
visceral pain 166–72
  cancer 128
  neurolytic blocks 65
  spinal cord injury 110, 111
visual analog scale (VAS) 34–5, 36

weight management 52, 140, 158
wide dynamic range neurons 17

ziconotide (SNX-111) 67

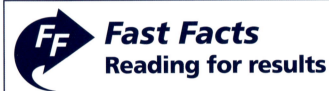

Fast Facts
Reading for results

Was this Fast Facts well worth reading?
Has it helped you make good health decisions?

Please post your comments in the box on the relevant page on **fastfacts.com**, and check out fellow readers' insights while you're there.

This is also the place to leave questions for the authors' consideration, and to spend 10 minutes on the free **FastTest** to ensure those key points really sunk in, and that you are set to apply them – **result!**

fastfacts.com